KAREN KAIN'S
FITNESS & BEAUTY
BOOK

For Ross,
who knows all the reasons why.

KAREN KAIN'S FITNESS & BEAUTY BOOK

As Told to Marilyn Linton

Photographs by Jim Allen

Doubleday Canada Limited, Toronto, Ontario
Doubleday & Company Inc., Garden City, New York
1983

Library of Congress Catalog Card Number: 82-46056

Copyright © 1983 by Karen Kain and Marilyn Linton
All rights reserved
First Edition

Printed and Bound in Canada by the John Deyell Company
Typeset by ART-U Graphics Ltd.

Jacket and Interior Design and Art Direction by David Wyman

Canadian Cataloguing in Publication Data

Kain, Karen, and Linton, Marilyn
Karen Kain's fitness and beauty book

ISBN 0-385-18854-4

1. Physical fitness for women.   2. Health.   3. Beauty,
Personal.   I. Linton, Marilyn.   II. Title.

RA781.K34   613.7′045   C83-098627-8

Contents

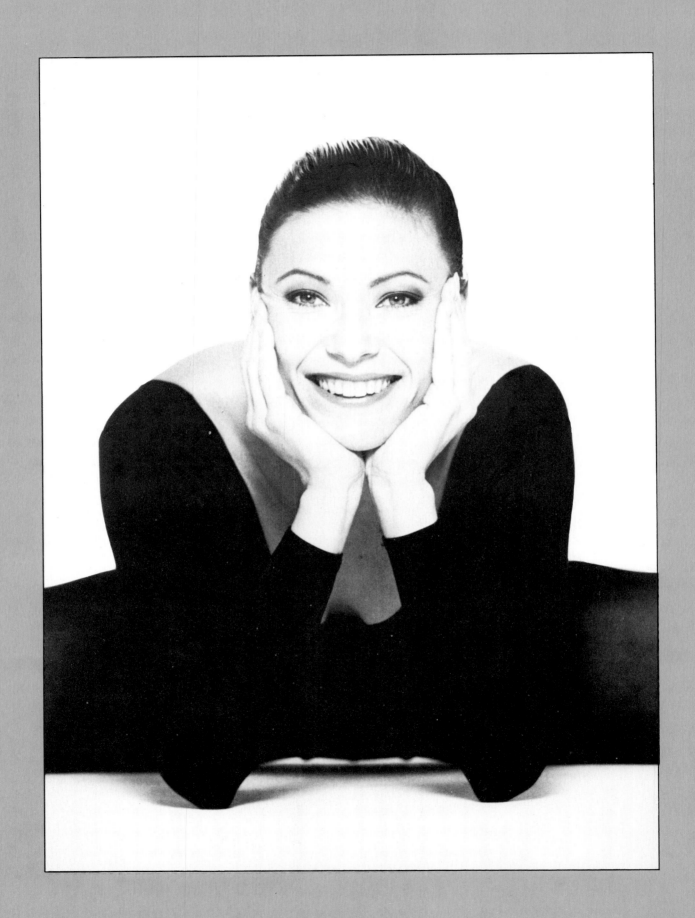

Introduction

Introduction

No project of this nature is undertaken without a purpose or message. There are two at work in this book.

The first is to clear away a misconception about those involved in ballet. The public can get carried away with the image of grace and control portrayed in a ballet production. There is a tendency to believe that the fluid forms that whirl and spin upon the stage just happen, that it is easy for those dancers to look fit and beautiful.

Unfortunately, that just isn't so. The coordination of many parts into a whole for even a single performance involves an incredible amount of strenuous work. Even those who have an appreciation of how hard it may be are misled if they believe that it is easy for a dancer to become and remain as fit as he or she appears on stage. We are creations of flesh and blood, subject to many of the same limitations as the people in the audience. Despite a dancer's slender form, it is wrong to assume that he or she naturally knows everything there is to know about fitness.

I have been involved in ballet since I was eight years old. At that age I never had to think about why I did the things my instructors taught me to do. I was simply told what to do because it was believed that tried and true methods properly prepared one for dancing. I followed the regimens set out and became fit, even though I did not always understand why I was doing certain moves.

Ballet is bound by tradition and fuelled by discipline. It combines the expression of art with the athletic ability required of an Olympic gymnast. In the realm of athletics, sport science and exercise physiology have developed for the systematic improvement of the athlete. Meanwhile, the practices prescribed for dancers have hardly changed since the 1800s, when some of the major works were created.

I cannot criticize the old methods too harshly, nor do I want to. Ballet is a big part of my life and I owe my success to the expert instructors and artistic traditions that I have followed for many, many years. However, when I was growing up and training to become a ballerina, I never really connected what I was doing with the fitness effect. When I became old enough to practice without instructors watching every minute, I found that I wasn't really sure what I should be doing to maintain total fitness. By the time I became an adult and took control of my life, I realized that I was not always going to be in shape, that I needed to learn a lot more in order to build and keep strength and stamina.

I started investigating, reading, talking to knowledgeable friends in the field of physical fitness, and seeking advice from my brother, Dr. Kevin Kain. To go with my newfound knowledge, I also had to develop self discipline to push myself when I needed it.

The results, in terms of my career, are self-evident. The ability to get through hundreds of practices and rehearsals, plus 35 demanding performances in a season is an important part of my life. Yet fitness goes far beyond that. While William Shakespeare observed that "all the world's a stage," I hasten to add that the stage does not make up all my world.

There *is* a vast world outside the ballet, and I love to enjoy it. Staying fit is the best insurance I have that there is enough energy left over to do just that. Herein lies the second message—one that is very real for every living soul.

The feeling of fitness can carry you into an unexplored dimension of yourself. You awake refreshed in the mornings to the sensual pleasure of feeling firm, toned muscles. You possess energy resources that have gone untapped since childhood, energy that carries you through the day. You have a heightened self-esteem in knowing that you look good. With this comes a new feeling of confidence and pride in knowing that you have committed yourself to improvement and really accomplished something. To use an automotive comparison, no one sees you travelling around town any more in a rusting jalopy. Instead, you're showing them the Rolls Royce that was always parked in your garage.

I know the difference, for I have been at the other end of the scale. There have been times when I've known that I haven't looked good in my clothes and rummaged through the closet to find something that covers properly, knowing that I couldn't wear a short skirt, finding that my waistbands were too tight. Fitness is something that I do for myself, and something I know you can do for yourself.

Beyond the psychological effects of fitness are, of course, the medical benefits. Diseases relating to the heart and circulatory system remain the biggest killers in North America. Doctors recognize the indications that regular exercise for cardiovascular fitness can reduce the risks for everyone and point the way to a longer, fuller life. Small wonder that many major corporations include membership in fitness clubs among the fringe benefits for their executives. With the potential of exercise to reduce stress and improve health, the companies are assuring themselves that their top people will be healthy, happy and productive for a longer time.

What follows is the distillation of what I have learned: a section on fitness in general to explain the importance and advantages of being in shape; a stimulating workout that will make you use and tone those muscles that will reshape the new you; a section on nutrition that will explain how you should nourish the body so that it can function properly, and how to alter your dietary habits for the better; a selection of my favorite recipes to help you make nutrition and diet a fun part of your life; sections on skin, hair, feet and hands with lots of tips on the right way to take care of them; and chapters on posture (with special back exercises), sleep and relaxation, to reduce stress and guide you to a brighter attitude towards life.

As they say when glasses are raised in celebration: "Here's to your health." It really is something to celebrate.

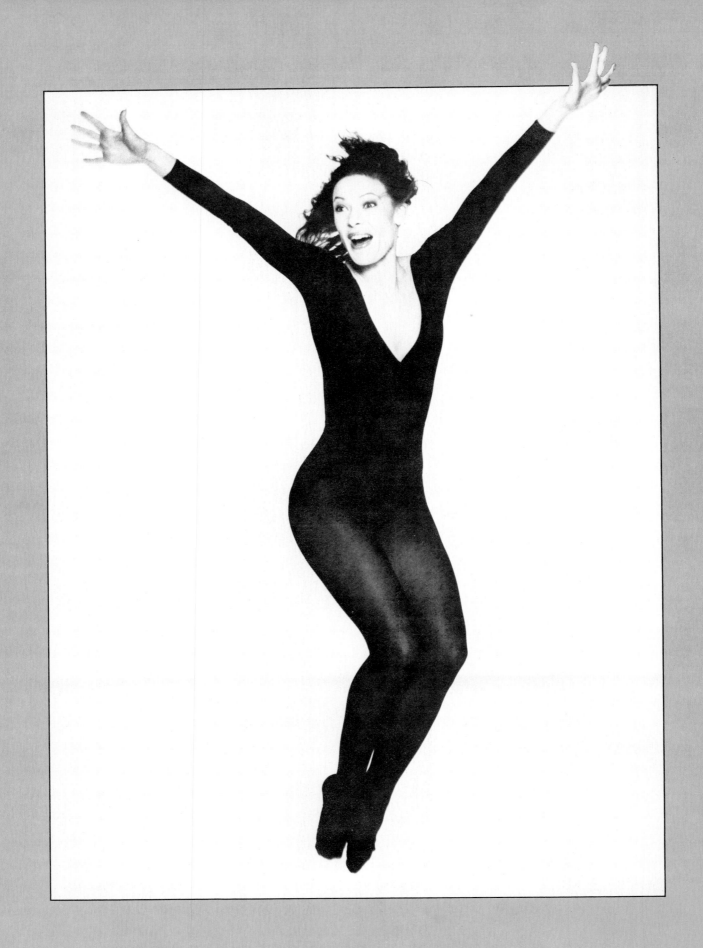

1

Fitness

Fitness

Fitness, in the most elementary sense of the word, means a suitability to a purpose. For the human body, that purpose is to see you through a full life. Your body is the vehicle in which you—the person—make that journey. The length, quality and enjoyment of life are all intimately related to the condition in which one maintains this marvellously engineered machine.

While the fitness industry continues to grow by leaps and bounds, it boggles the mind that so many people still neglect personal fitness. Science tells us that by looking after ourselves we improve our chances of avoiding heart disease, which remains the biggest killer in North America. Regular exercise for cardiovascular fitness is the key. It is the one way we can have a direct effect on several factors that have been directly connected to heart problems and stroke. We *can* retard the process of arteriosclerosis (the clogging of veins and arteries) so that we are not as susceptible to untimely death.

Arteriosclerosis begins at a very young age if diet and activity levels are not right. Young babies, who have died when no more than two years old, have been found to have a buildup of cholesterol plaques in the aorta of the heart. Fifty percent of the soldiers autopsied after dying in the Korean War—20-year olds who should have been in the prime of life—were found to have had their arteries narrowed from 50 to 75 percent.

I am exceptionally lucky in that I have a personal advisor in medical matters who can keep me updated on what happens in the world of physical fitness and how it affects my health. I have the utmost respect for Dr. Kevin Kain, my brother.

It is said that those who are closest to us are best suited to impart lasting and meaningful information that will affect our lives. If we have a problem that is not visible to ourselves or that we deny when everyone else notices, these important people have a way of coming through to give us the straight goods. In this regard, I say "thank heaven for little brothers." Much of what follows is information which he has shared with me—for my own good and now for yours.

Science stresses cardiovascular fitness above all when it comes to preventive medicine. The heart and lungs are the organs that provide the oxygen to the body's tissues so that we can convert what we eat into energy. The better they are conditioned, the easier their task. This is measured by a number that tells you how efficiently the body is using the oxygen supplied. The number is referred to in sport and fitness as VO_2 max, for the maximum volume of oxygen taken up by the body, per kilogram of body mass, per minute of activity.

At the time of many professional sport training camps, you may have seen pictures in daily newspapers of athletes on a stationary bicycle (ergometer) or on a treadmill, with masks attached to their faces to collect the gasses exhaled. This is a common method of measuring VO_2 max. It is also done at most of the major fitness clubs as part of a fitness inventory.

Generally speaking, aerobic activities, such as jogging, swimming, cycling and cross-country skiing, improve one's rating in VO_2 max because respiration or air intake increases, and the heart pumps oxygen-rich blood harder for some length of time. As more oxygen becomes available to the muscles used during exercise, their ability to consume oxygen for energy increases.

The VO_2 max figure for some top athletes is quite high. While the resting VO_2 max is pegged at about 3.5 millilitres of oxygen per kilogram of weight per minute of activity, it has been measured in the range of 80 to 85 ml/kg/min for elite marathon runners, whose bodies function as finely tuned machines. The slight edge goes to the skiers because they use their arms as well as their legs for propulsion. The larger the muscle mass used, the greater the body's total consumption of oxygen.

The figures compare with a shockingly low average of about 42 km/kg/min for the average college-age man. The figure is lower still for women of a similar age and activity level. By the time women reach the age of 30, the average VO_2 max can be down to 25. Women tend to have a VO_2 max between 10 and 15 percent lower than men on the average. The reasons are not entirely clear, although some of it may have to do with the extra sex-specific fat that women carry (we can't do anything about it), or their lower haemoglobin level. Yet even when VO_2 max is measured in terms of lean body mass (fat tissues excluded) the difference between sexes does not disappear entirely.

The measurement of VO_2 max is considered highly stable. The time of day at which the test is taken, donation of a pint of blood, prolonged loss of sleep and repeating the procedure with very little time between tests have all been found *not* to influence the measurement of VO_2 max significantly. You can feel tired and wretched, but the VO_2 max will not reflect that. It is useful to science in that it is an objective, rather than a subjective measure. For those who are not already involved in some kind of aerobic program to improve cardiovascular fitness, the undertaking of a fitness regimen can produce an increase of 10 percent in VO_2 max over a ten-week period. You know your exercise program is doing something for you when your VO_2 max goes up.

Aerobic exercise is that which uses oxygen over a long period of time. Conversely, anaerobic activity usually refers to exercise or activity that is done in short bursts. The way to get an idea of whether or not you are working aerobically is through monitoring your own heart rate via the pulse. You should aim for a target zone in terms of the number of times your heart beats per minute. Determining that target zone can be done by an easy rule of thumb. The upper limit of heartbeats per minute is 200 minus your age; the lower limit is 170 minus your age. Take your pulse a few minutes into the workout.

The pulse can be taken at the wrist, by gently pressing two fingers next to the tendon that is visible when you form a loose fist. It can also be taken in the throat area, by pressing lightly again with two fingers next to the Adam's apple. Don't try to measure for a full minute because the pulse rate will drop off as you cool down. It is better to count the number of beats in 10 seconds and multiply that figure by six or the number in 15 seconds and multiply by four. This gives a more accurate measure of your heart rate during exercise, so that you know whether to increase your intensity or to slack off to get back into the target zone.

To achieve a fitness effect, you should spend at least 20 minutes, three times a week with your heart in the target zone. This is a minimum. It is far wiser to make exercise part of your regular daily regimen. Let it become part of your routine, so that you feel the day is incomplete or that you've cheated yourself out of a good feeling if you haven't worked out.

For some, the workout included in this book will be enough of an aerobic activity at the start if you flow from one exercise into another. However, as you progress, it will become apparent that the exercises are geared more toward flexibility, stretching and toning the muscles that will help reshape you. Physically advanced readers are urged to take on some form of aerobic activity—brisk walking, jogging, skipping—in conjunction with this workout. The exercises are still valid for them, but they may be more useful for warming up and cooling down.

Keeping the heart healthy cannot be stressed enough. In the United States alone, there are approximately one million heart attacks each year and about 60 percent of the victims die. While we tend to think of a heart attack as a very sudden occurrence, the fact is that in most cases there has been damage in progress for a long period of time. Doctors point to a number of risk factors along the cardiac trail. Some of them, we cannot alter; others we can.

One's age, sex and family history won't change no matter how much exercise you do. The longer you've lived, the more opportunity there is for arteriosclerosis to take place and clog arteries. Hormonal differences and an historic tendency for men to be subjected to stress in the workplace (though this is changing) have led to men having a higher risk of cardiovascular complications than women. While family history may indicate a predisposition to heart failure through some genetically originated malfunction, a good fitness program can still ward off other contributing factors to heart disease. Even if half your family died at a young age with heart problems, exercise will give you the best possible chance to live out a full life.

High blood pressure, another of the primary risk factors, is modifiable. There is an opportunity to control high blood pressure and hypertension through diet, exercise, stress management and medication. Likewise, high cholesterol levels can be governed by diet and workouts. There are two different carriers of cholesterol in the blood, identified as HDL (high density lipoproteins) and LDL (low density lipoproteins).

In simple terms, you want to have more HDL than LDL. High density lipoprotein cholesterol is believed to carry cholesterol away from the walls of the arteries and into the liver, where it is destroyed. It can be termed cardio-protective. The level of HDL goes up with the amount of exercise done. It has a function of cleaning up the circulatory system, while LDL has been identified with the clogging process. The risk of having too much LDL can be reduced by reducing the intake of animal fats and the ratio between the two can be changed through exercise.

Another active way of reducing the risk of heart problems is to stop smoking. Smokers run a risk between two and six times greater than non-smokers of having heart disease. Nicotine has been shown to cause constriction of the blood vessels, while at the same time elevating the heart rate. This causes the blood pressure to leap.

Furthermore, when you take in the smoke from these expensive burning leaves in a paper tube, you are taking in carbon monoxide, rather than oxygen. You reduce the oxygen-carrying capacity of the blood and make the heart work very hard to make up the shortfall in oxygen supply. The good news is that the risks do come back down once a smoker has sworn off the habit.

Obesity, or being overweight, is another factor adding to the risk of cardiovascular disease. Did you know that every extra pound of fat in the body requires a full mile of blood vessels? That's quite an amount of extra work to place upon the heart. My brother Kevin tells me of a lady who was hospitalized when she was 100 pounds overweight. Someone walked in and told her about all the extra miles of blood vessels she had—not very subtly. "Keep going lady. You're halfway to Montreal!"

There are, of course, other medical benefits to be derived from exercise. The Type A personality, the outgoing, intense, take-it-all-seriously, my-world-ends-in-five-minutes people of this world put themselves under a great deal of stress and drive up their chances of heart attack, along with their blood pressure, by constricting blood vessels. Exercise gives them the opportunity to ventilate their emotion and hostility. Vigorous exercise can also release a substance into the body known as endorphin—it is a natural sedative.

Even diabetics, who have a high risk of circulatory disease because excess glucose collects in arterioles, can be helped by exercise. It has been shown that exercise can drive blood sugar into bodily tissue where it can be burned off.

This is all preventive medicine. Canada and the United States have huge bills for intensive care units and rehabilitative units that are filled with people who don't have to be there—at least not if they had looked after themselves. It costs us all too much in both human and financial resources.

All it takes is a few minutes a day to improve your health. It can be done so easily—even to music. Find a song with a good beat, something that gets you going, that you can hum along to. It helps the time pass and takes your mind off the fact that this is something like work. Or jump on a exercise bike in front of your favorite television show. Open a window wide so that you have plenty of fresh air and oxygen to feed the muscles, and go for it.

Which Exercises?

The selection of an aerobic activity to complement your workout program is a highly individualistic matter. True, you want to take on something that will serve the dual purpose of building the cardiovascular system while burning off excess calories. However, not everyone is suited to attempt the more demanding activities, at least not at the start.

This is another case where you should let your doctor give you some advice about how much to undertake. While cardiovascular-oriented activities are meant to give you stamina, you already need a certain degree of fitness to handle some of them. The person who has led a sedentary existence since school days would be ill-advised to throw himself whole-heartedly into running when jogging or brisk walking can accomplish the same thing.

Remember that to get aerobic conditioning effects, it is necessary to raise the heart rate into the target zone and keep it there for at least 20 minutes, a minimum of three times per week.

While it is hardly a good thing to be out of shape, it may come as some consolation that those who are out of shape don't need to do as much to raise their heart rates. Carrying around extra weight can make a brisk walk just as strenuous for some as a flat-out run. In cases such as these, there is little trouble in making the time for exercise. Leave a little early for work and, instead of fighting for a parking space near the office, park the car a mile away and hoof it. If you take mass transit, get off the subway or bus a few stops early. It's a great way to make cardiovascular exercise a part of your routine.

It is also a way to get the edge on the battle against calories. By the time you reach work, you'll have already burned off breakfast. Weight loss or gain is a simple matter of addition or subtraction: take in more calories than you burn off in a day and you are adding fat; use more calories than you consume, and you are on your way to a trimmer, sleeker figure. One pound of fat is equivalent to about 3,500 calories, so that a sensible diet—not a crash diet or starvation diet—combined with increased activity means weight loss.

As your cardiovascular system becomes stronger, your lungs are able to process more oxygen and the heart is able to do more work with fewer beats. Your blood vessels regain some of their suppleness and that facilitates blood flow. Some of the good endurance exercises, aside from running, jogging or brisk walking, include swimming, skipping rope, cycling, athletic dancing, cross-country skiing and recreation sports that require constant activity, such as soccer, basketball, racquetball, squash, badminton and tennis. (The racquet sports will only do you good if you are playing against someone who is competitive at your level. It does you no good to stand and watch your opponent's passing shots all day.)

The true beauty about aerobic activities and cardiovascular fitness is the variety of exercises that can be done either alone or with a group. You may have your favorites among them, but it is also wonderful to know that you can switch off to another sport to break the tedium if one particular activity becomes boring.

Walking

The brisk walking that we mentioned earlier can consume 160 calories in 30 minutes. It is an activity that comes highly recommended by doctors and exercise physiologists because, unlike running and jogging, it places little stress on the ankle and knee joints while at the same time it requires that the heart and lungs deliver oxygenated blood to some of the largest muscles in the body. It tones the leg muscles (and an exceptionally long stride can help firm up the buttocks).

Wear comfortable shoes and walk with a slight spring to the step, rolling from the heel to the ball of the foot. Two thin pairs of socks are advised to prevent blisters. Be systematic and set out a course, to and from the house or office. As your level of fitness increases, vary the course to add some uphill walking or progress to jogging or running if you believe (and your doctor must agree) your joints and back can handle it.

Jogging

Jogging, gentler and slower than running, burns off about 300 calories per half-hour. Properly cushioned shoes help take some of the jolt out of running on pavement. Many sport supply stores also carry what is known as a jogging bra for women.

Gravity and the passage of time do enough to a woman's breasts without the added effects of the jogger's bouncy gait. A proper jogging bra can also ward off a condition known as jogger's nipple, caused when that same motion makes the tender tissue chafe against the runner's blouse or singlet.

As with brisk walking, build up your endurance gradually by making the course more difficult or increasing the length of the activity.

Running

Most of the things said already about walking and jogging also apply to running, which burns off some 425 calories per half-hour. This aerobic venture, however, should be saved for a more advanced level of fitness and one must always be aware of bodily signs that running is taking a toll on the joints or back. It may be wise to alternate running with walking and jogging to give the body some chance to adjust.

Skipping

Good, old-fashioned skipping is an activity that often gets overlooked when people think of exercise, yet it can burn 400 calories per half-hour and is an excellent substitute for running in inclement weather or late at night, when you may not feel safe taking to the streets.

Don't feel sheepish about going back to a childhood activity. Boxers have used skipping ropes for generations as one of the best methods of building up calf muscles in the lower leg and increasing the body's stamina. A simple piece of rope and a little clear space are all you need. It's an excellent activity to do to music or while watching the television to keep your mind off the boredom that may come with the repetitive nature of the exercise.

Cross-Country Skiing

A winter substitute for running or jogging is cross-country skiing, which is growing rapidly in popularity. Done at a high level, this can burn off some 500 calories per half-hour because the legs and arms, too, are used for propulsion. The sliding motion of the skis is easier on the knees than the run on pavement. There are trails across every province and territory of Canada and most of them rent equipment and provide lessons for beginners. It is not difficult to get a feel for the sport and the winter scenery can be spectacular. Protect yourself from the cold with a few thin layers that allow mobility, rather than a single thick covering.

Swimming

It will please the overweight people of this world to know that fat floats. The more overweight you are, the greater your buoyancy is apt to be. Many people find that when they come back to swimming later in life, it is easier than they remembered. Swimming can burn some 260 calories per half-hour and provides a tremendous workout for muscles in the arms, shoulders and back. Most towns with municipal pools provide convenient public swimming times, summer and winter.

Cycling

Besides being an alternative method of pollution-free transportation, cycling consumes about 130 calories per half-hour, providing you don't ride downhill, coasting all the way. A stationary exercise bike can provide even more exercise because the tension with which you pedal is adjustable.

You do not need a fancy 10- or 12-speed bike to get aerobic benefits. A second-hand bicycle will do all you want in terms of exercising the legs and re-establishing a good sense of balance. The seat may cause a little soreness at first, but this will pass in about a week if you bike regularly. As with swimming, because the body weight is supported, the knees are somewhat protected. You shouldn't do any cartilage damage, although the ligaments and muscles will get a workout.

Racquet Sports

I mentioned that racquet sports are another good aerobic alternative if played with someone competitive at your level so that there is constant flow and motion in the game. Tennis is estimated to use about 220 calories per half-hour and squash and racquetball some 300. While the activity and social aspects are highly desirable, there is this caveat—playing regularly can become expensive because it could require membership in a private club or payment of court costs or both. Add in the costs of court shoes, racquets and eye-protectors and you have made something of an investment in the fitness business.

Dancersizing

I would be remiss if I didn't include dancing or dancersize as it is called, among aerobic activities. Depending on the degree of athletics you throw into dancing, you can burn anywhere from 200 to 300 calories an hour. Styles can range anywhere from tap dance, which stresses work at the legs and ankles, to the full-body workout supplied by jazz dance and gymnastic floor exercise.

Aside from the benefits to your heart and lungs, your co-ordination, suppleness and flexibility will also improve with dancing. Leotards, leg warmers and slippers may be all the equipment you require. It is a form of exercise that can be taken up at any age, at any degree of difficulty suited to the dancer—and with almost any ethnic flavor he or she desires.

Certainly there are the modern, packaged dance tapes and records; but more traditional dances have their place in the muscle workout. Spanish flamenco works the calves and the backs of the legs and buttocks; Hawaiian hula works the hips into flexibility; the belly dances of the East provide a tremendous workout for the abdomen and back. Even a long polka can raise the heart rate to where you want it for cardiovascular development.

Most of all, dance can prove to be the most fun and most varied of all the aerobic activities. It can be done alone, with a partner, to music and to moonlight. Some people would even choose to make a career of dance. We won't name names.

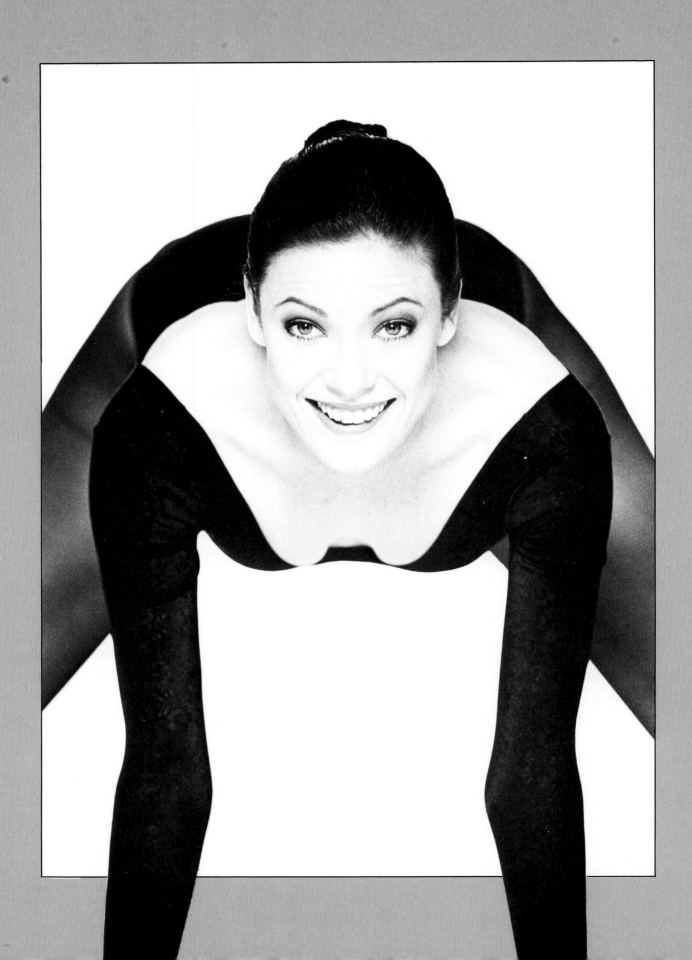

2

The Karen Kain Workout

The Karen Kain Workout

I mentioned earlier in this book that two of the fabulous fringe benefits of becoming fit are the way your new body looks and the way it makes you feel. You're not only gift-wrapping the person you are and maximizing your attractiveness, but in the mornings you spring to your feet rather than tumble out of bed, ready to face and conquer the challenges of the day.

There are two different types of exercise. The new look comes from exercises that tone the muscles to reshape you. The feeling of fitness and energy comes from training the cardiovascular system and consequently increasing your energy reserve and ability to use oxygen. This is what I meant in my earlier discussion of aerobic activity. It's worth it to you and it can be accomplished in as little as 30 minutes a day.

I advise one thing before taking on any exercise or diet program. Please consult your doctor first and let him know what you intend to do—what your goals are and what your method will be for attaining those goals. Chances are the doctor will applaud your attitude and initiative (even though staying fit is a good form of preventive medicine and deprives him of some income; he and his wallet will be seeing less of you, in more ways than one).

However, he may also give you some important guidelines, particular to your body because he knows it from the inside out. Your doctor is the best person to determine what you can take on without unduly stressing your heart or various parts of your body. For instance, people with unstable lower backs may be advised against particular exercises such as toe-touching from a standing position, or leg lifts from a laying position. He might warn against starting out with too much emphasis on the arms, since the heart is sometimes required to pump harder to get blood through veins and capillaries that are smaller than those in the legs. The doctor can suggest alternative exercises to work the same muscles, while reducing the risk of injury. Allow your doctor to advise you as to the rate and intensity at which you undertake your program.

The workout that I have put together for this book is geared primarily at reshaping the figure through toning the muscles. If you are not accustomed to working out, it may also raise your heart rate into the target zone so that you derive some aerobic benefit as well. This will be the case especially once you have learned the exercise sequences well enough to move from one into the next, with very little break in between. The workout has been organized specifically to permit this sort of flow in the movement. The workout alone may be sufficient daily exercise for the beginner.

However, I would advise using these exercises in conjunction with a program of walking, jogging, biking, swimming, jazz dancing or some other form of sustained aerobic activity. As you progress and as your general fitness level increases, the toning and shaping workout will maintain its importance for those specific purposes, although it won't be doing as much for your aerobic capacity. It should remain incorporated as a warm-up and cool-down phase of your other daily activities.

I stress daily, because to maintain or improve your level of cardiovascular fitness and to maintain body shape, fitness ought to become a habit. While exercise physiologists tell us that a fitness effect can be achieved with as little as 20 minutes of work in the heart target zone, three times a week, I'd recommend more than that, for two reasons. The first, obviously, is that you will begin seeing and feeling the encouraging results much more quickly. The second is that daily repetition will rapidly make it part of your regular routine. If you can get into the habit of doing something six or seven times a week, you'll develop a feeling of guilt that you are cheating yourself if you have a lazy day when you have trouble being motivated to work out. Resenting your own laziness may give you the impetus you need.

A few suggestions before your first crack at the workout. Have a look at what is called the pelvic tilt, a simple movement that puts the spine in alignment. Not only is the pelvic tilt part of the remedy for bad posture, but it is necessary for some exercises involving the abdominal muscles because it can direct strain away from the delicate lower back. Second, take notice that there are different numbers of repetitions of each move prescribed for beginners and advanced exercisers. Don't try to overdo a particular move in your first few attempts. Read the instructions carefully and try to execute the moves as accurately as possible to get the full benefit from them. Feel the appropriate muscles at work. Certainly you can't expect to copy my examples in the accompanying pictures exactly, especially in the stretches. My muscles and joints have been doing some of these moves since I was eight years old. However, you can aim to look like the pictures as a long-range goal.

You will notice as well that there are seven additional exercises labelled the Tough-it-Out Seven. These are meant for advanced practitioners and should be inserted just before the wind-down phase when you have reached the stage that you feel you can handle a little more work. Don't forget to follow them up with the wind-down.

Listen to your body and take care of it. You can grit your teeth to get through a little pain and strain, but be aware of the source of the problem. A little stiffness in the muscles can be expected, but if pain persists—particularly back pain—check with your doctor again.

Toning of various muscle groups does much to shape the body. Take the problem of the pot belly. Even people who don't carry a lot of fatty tissue can have this problem. One reason it can happen is that the abdominal muscles are poorly toned. When this occurs, the mere weight of the intestines and internal organs causes the tummy to bulge forward and give you roundness where you want it least. There isn't sufficient strong muscle tissue to hold them back in place. Tightening the abdominal muscles has the effect of supplying you with a built-in girdle, like walking around with your tummy held in all the time. At the same time, the back can derive some benefit from the exercises that you use to strengthen the abdomen. Many lower back problems crop up because of weak abdominal muscles.

The remaining points I want to make about exercise and this workout concern the fact that it doesn't have to feel like drudgery. Even though you realize you are doing something good for yourself, when you start out and feel a few aches and pains from muscles that haven't been worked in a long time, it can seem easy to give up and declare your personal salvage project to be a total loss.

Don't do anything of the kind.

Part of those aches and pains can be eliminated by making sure you do the proper stretches found at the beginning and end of the workout and interspersed throughout it. It is imperative that when you work a muscle hard, you stretch it out. All athletes appreciate this—even four-legged athletes. At race tracks, when a horse has finished running a race, it is not simply led back to its stall. If this happened, the horse's muscles would stiffen up and the owner would have a lame animal on his hands. Instead, at the end of the race, a young stablehand, known as a hot-walker, takes the horse and keeps him pacing up and down shedrow until the muscles have had ample time to cool down slowly.

Likewise, when a runner wins the 1,500-metre race at the Olympics, he doesn't stop dead and take a bow. He takes a victory lap and does hurdler's stretches. Swimmers repair to the warm-up pool to "warm-down."

A good deal of muscle soreness occurs because there is a buildup of lactic acid in the muscle tissue when you do hard work. This happens especially when you do some anaerobic activity such as sprinting or, in dancing, a strenuous *pas de deux*. Dr. Kevin Kain identifies this as anaerobic glycolysis, as the muscles begin to burn without enough oxygen being supplied. A sprinter hardly has time to draw in enough air to meet the workload he is doing. In our workout, let's make sure we remember to keep breathing deeply.

If your soreness is coming from a buildup of lactic acid, you can get rid of that lactate by increasing blood flow to the muscles—stretching and winding down.

It seems curious to me that although ballet dancers recognize the value of this type of stretching after their morning classes and rehearsals, they often forget about it at 11 P.M., when an equally demanding performance has been completed. For too many of us, the day's work is done and we hastily change out of our costumes and head off home or to a party. Inevitably, it takes most of the next morning to get the kinks out, even for well-conditioned dancers.

I find that for myself, a whirlpool bath or a massage will have approximately the same effect as stretching because circulation is stimulated within the muscles. A sauna will not do the job. What a sauna or steam bath does is raise the skin temperature and increase the heart rate, whereas the effect you want is to cool down slowly from the inside out. Not everyone can afford the luxuries of having a massage or whirlpool, but "walking it out" can be equally effective—and considerably less expensive.

By avoiding muscle soreness, you'll find yourself much more willing, and capable, to follow up the next day, and the next.

Another way of making the workout more enjoyable is to do it where there is a lot of air and open space. I have mentioned before the role of oxygen in building aerobic capacity (VO_2 max) and how an oxygen debt can lead to lactic acid buildup and sore muscles. Why not take your summer workouts out of doors, where you can let your muscles feast on oxygen. If you must be a captive of four walls, then have a fan blowing to keep the air circulating. Remember to breathe deeply.

Music is a tremendous boon in taking the tedium out of exercise as well. I mentioned before that although I am fond of the classics, they are not always suited to vigorous workouts. I found a compromise. Not long ago, some musical arranger made a hatful of cash and did athletic music fans a huge favor by setting classics to a turned-on, driving disco beat. In fact I suspect that because disco lends itself so easily to exercise programs, it can be given part of the credit for the boom in the fitness business with the proliferation of "dancersize" classes, albums and tapes.

It's certainly more pleasant than listening to the type of martial music that used to be associated with physical education classes. Actually, any type of music that is pleasing to the ear can be incorporated in the workout. Make sure it is lively and rhythmic enough to inspire activity. You can go to something more mellow for the stretches.

One last tip. I have found that the careful use of weight training can accelerate the process of muscle toning. The muscles are required to do more work because they are operating against more resistance than the weight of your own limbs or body. Fewer repetitions are required for muscles to achieve the same workload and shaping can take place faster. Women need not put on the same sort of muscle bulk that men do.

Bear two things in mind, however. Weight training should only be done under the supervision of a qualified instructor. Secondly, weight training is not a cardiovascular activity and cannot replace a good run when it comes to aerobic fitness. Weights fall into the toning and shaping category and you should not let your heart and lungs suffer by doing this to the exclusion of aerobic activities.

The Warm-Up

1. Head Rolls

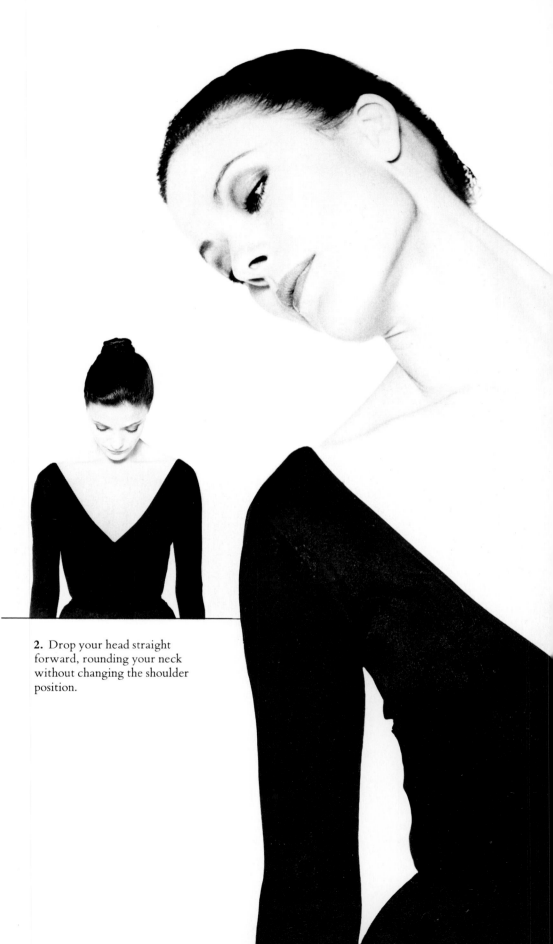

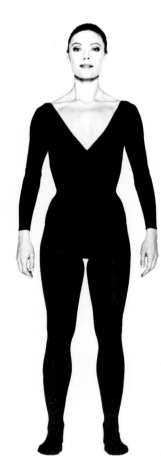

1. Stand with your arms relaxed at your sides, feet slightly apart. Pull in your tummy and squeeze your buttocks.

2. Drop your head straight forward, rounding your neck without changing the shoulder position.

3. Rotate your head to the right, feeling the stretch on the left side of your neck. Don't bunch up your shoulders.

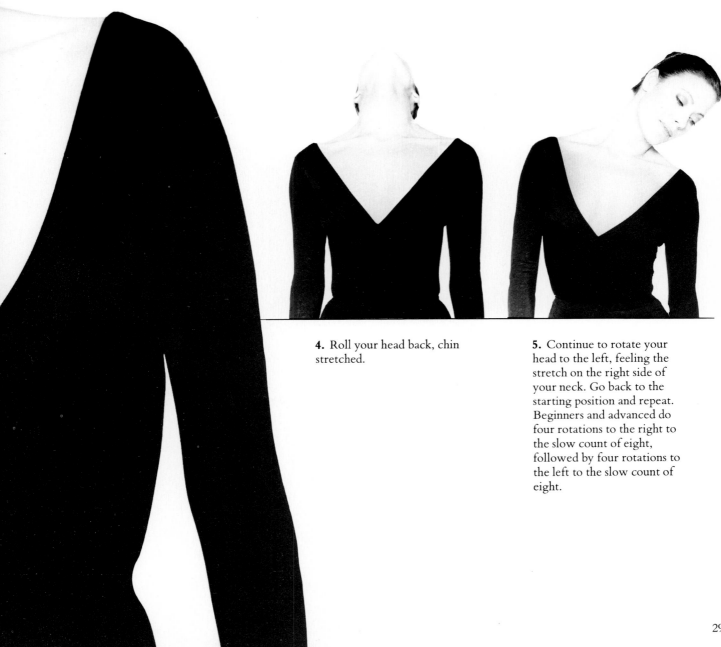

4. Roll your head back, chin stretched.

5. Continue to rotate your head to the left, feeling the stretch on the right side of your neck. Go back to the starting position and repeat. Beginners and advanced do four rotations to the right to the slow count of eight, followed by four rotations to the left to the slow count of eight.

THE WARM-UP

2. Shoulder Lift 'n' Roll

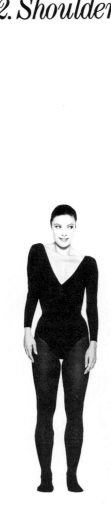

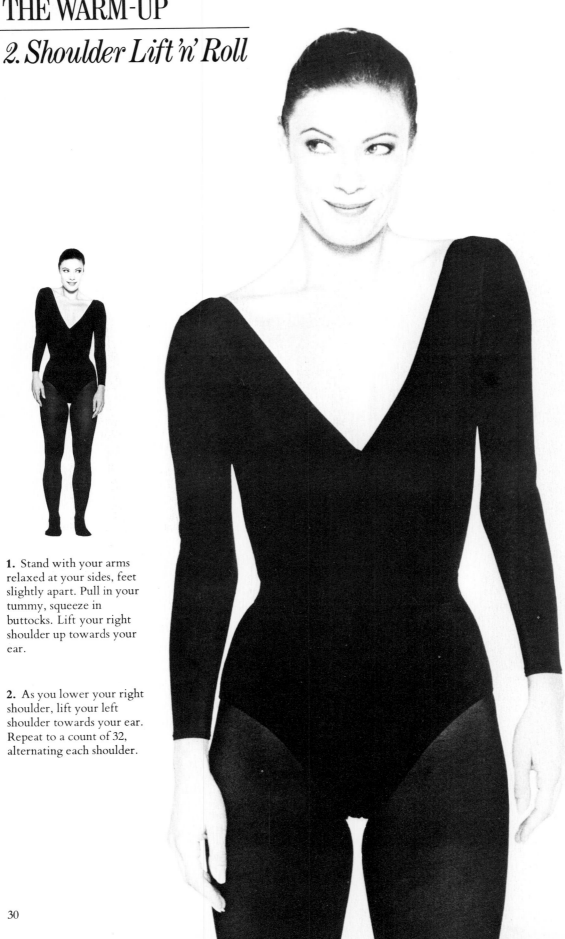

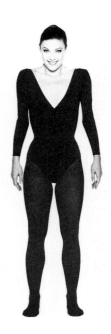

1. Stand with your arms relaxed at your sides, feet slightly apart. Pull in your tummy, squeeze in buttocks. Lift your right shoulder up towards your ear.

2. As you lower your right shoulder, lift your left shoulder towards your ear. Repeat to a count of 32, alternating each shoulder.

3. Next, move both shoulders in a circular motion. Do this eight times forward and eight times backward.

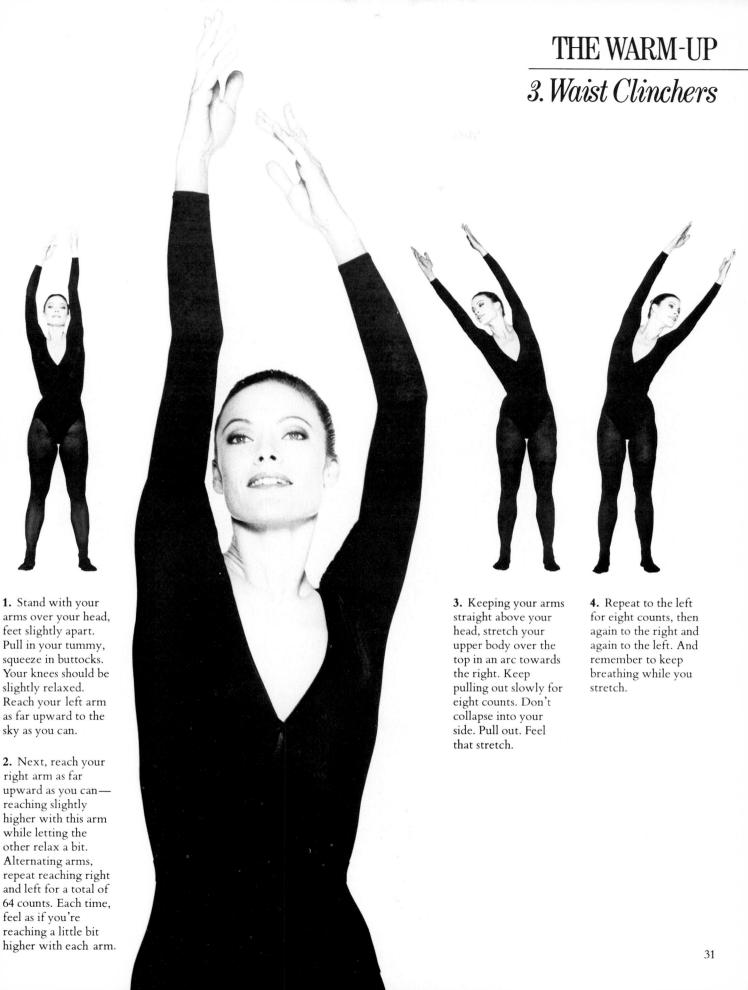

1. Stand with your arms over your head, feet slightly apart. Pull in your tummy, squeeze in buttocks. Your knees should be slightly relaxed. Reach your left arm as far upward to the sky as you can.

2. Next, reach your right arm as far upward as you can—reaching slightly higher with this arm while letting the other relax a bit. Alternating arms, repeat reaching right and left for a total of 64 counts. Each time, feel as if you're reaching a little bit higher with each arm.

3. Keeping your arms straight above your head, stretch your upper body over the top in an arc towards the right. Keep pulling out slowly for eight counts. Don't collapse into your side. Pull out. Feel that stretch.

4. Repeat to the left for eight counts, then again to the right and again to the left. And remember to keep breathing while you stretch.

31

4. The Waist Twist

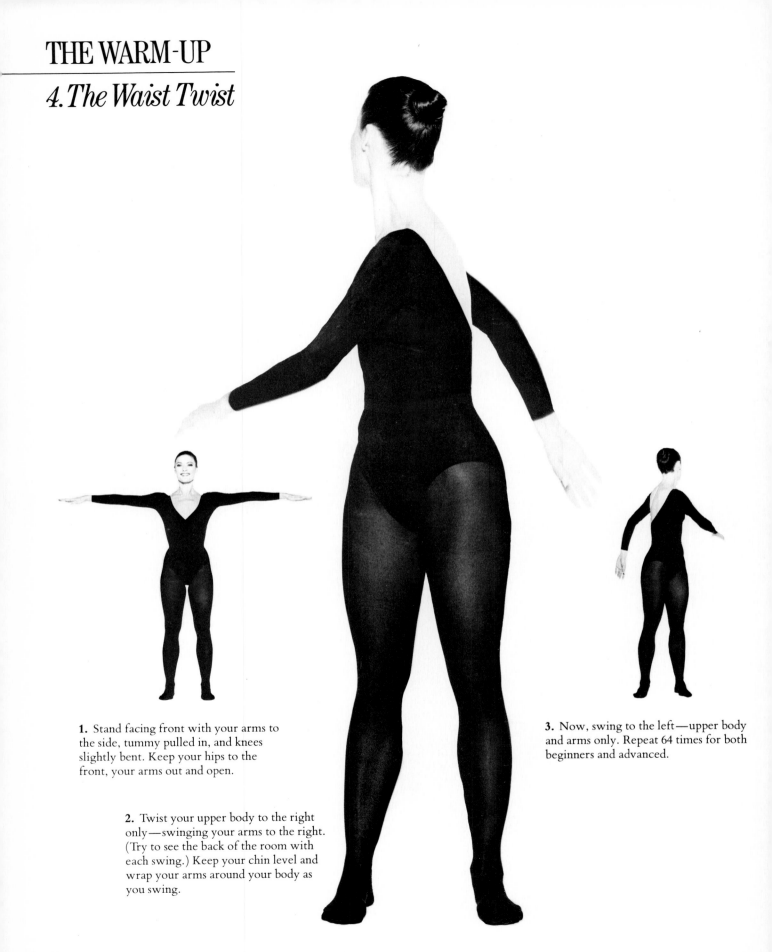

1. Stand facing front with your arms to the side, tummy pulled in, and knees slightly bent. Keep your hips to the front, your arms out and open.

2. Twist your upper body to the right only—swinging your arms to the right. (Try to see the back of the room with each swing.) Keep your chin level and wrap your arms around your body as you swing.

3. Now, swing to the left—upper body and arms only. Repeat 64 times for both beginners and advanced.

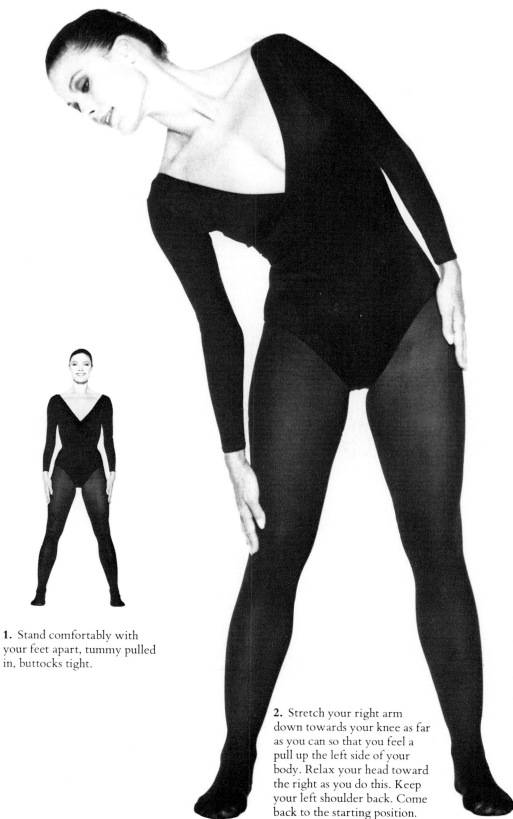

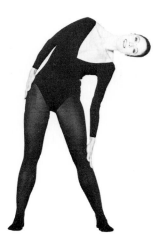

1. Stand comfortably with your feet apart, tummy pulled in, buttocks tight.

2. Stretch your right arm down towards your knee as far as you can so that you feel a pull up the left side of your body. Relax your head toward the right as you do this. Keep your left shoulder back. Come back to the starting position.

3. Repeat exercise to the left. Repeat the entire exercise 32 times on each side for beginners, and 64 times for advanced—alternating sides.

6. The Runner's Stretch

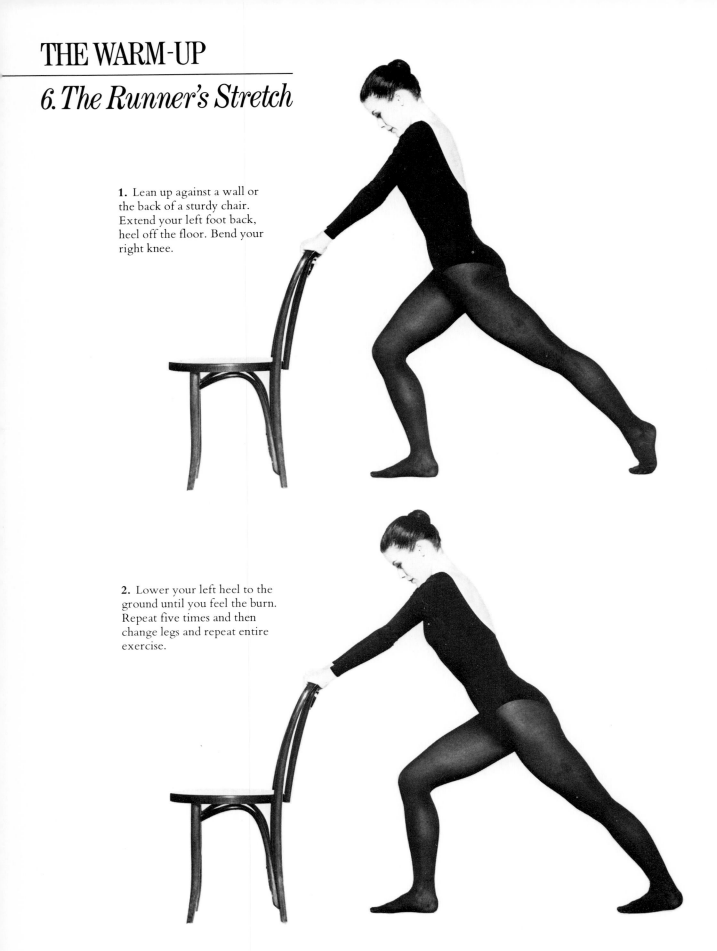

1. Lean up against a wall or the back of a sturdy chair. Extend your left foot back, heel off the floor. Bend your right knee.

2. Lower your left heel to the ground until you feel the burn. Repeat five times and then change legs and repeat entire exercise.

The Workout

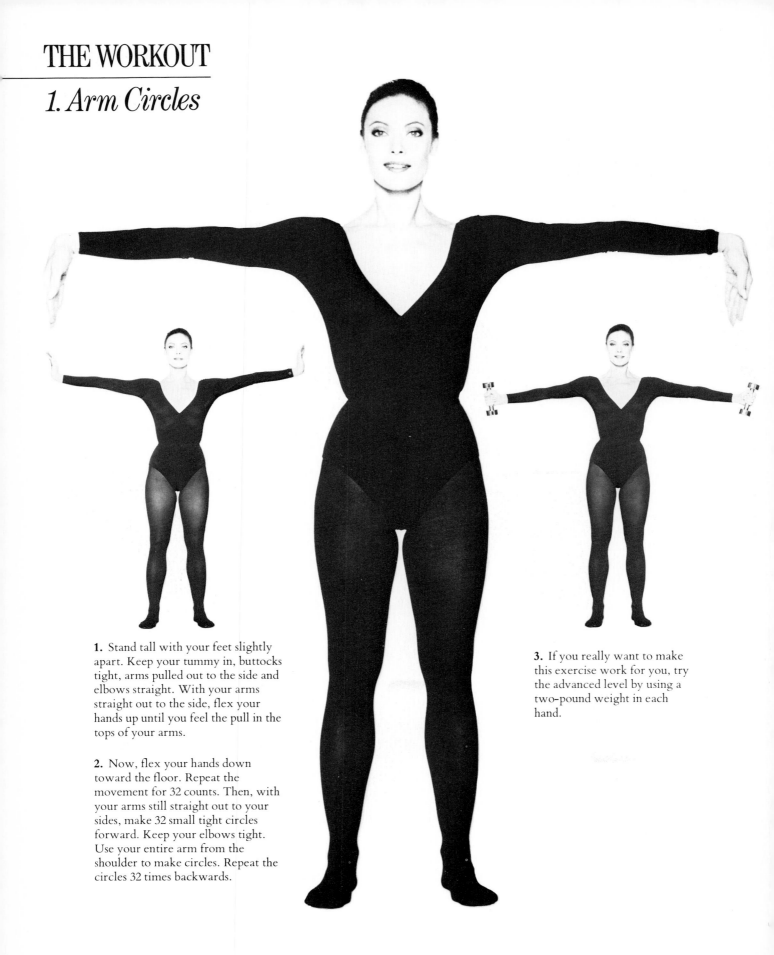

THE WORKOUT
1. Arm Circles

1. Stand tall with your feet slightly apart. Keep your tummy in, buttocks tight, arms pulled out to the side and elbows straight. With your arms straight out to the side, flex your hands up until you feel the pull in the tops of your arms.

2. Now, flex your hands down toward the floor. Repeat the movement for 32 counts. Then, with your arms still straight out to your sides, make 32 small tight circles forward. Keep your elbows tight. Use your entire arm from the shoulder to make circles. Repeat the circles 32 times backwards.

3. If you really want to make this exercise work for you, try the advanced level by using a two-pound weight in each hand.

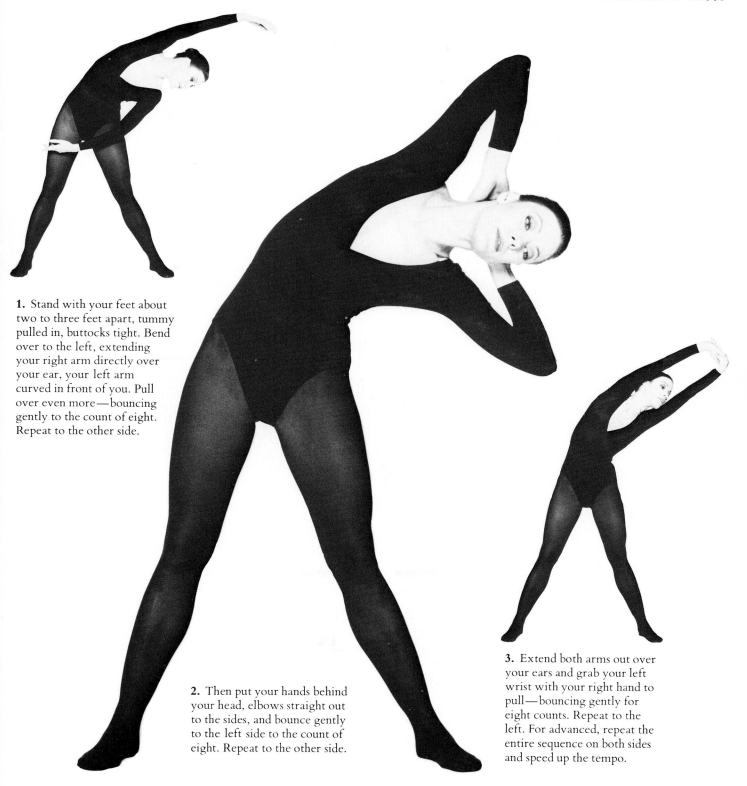

1. Stand with your feet about two to three feet apart, tummy pulled in, buttocks tight. Bend over to the left, extending your right arm directly over your ear, your left arm curved in front of you. Pull over even more—bouncing gently to the count of eight. Repeat to the other side.

2. Then put your hands behind your head, elbows straight out to the sides, and bounce gently to the left side to the count of eight. Repeat to the other side.

3. Extend both arms out over your ears and grab your left wrist with your right hand to pull—bouncing gently for eight counts. Repeat to the left. For advanced, repeat the entire sequence on both sides and speed up the tempo.

THE WORKOUT
Ballet-The First Position

The next five exercises are all used in a ballet dancer's daily workout. They begin with this position, known as "first position" in ballet.

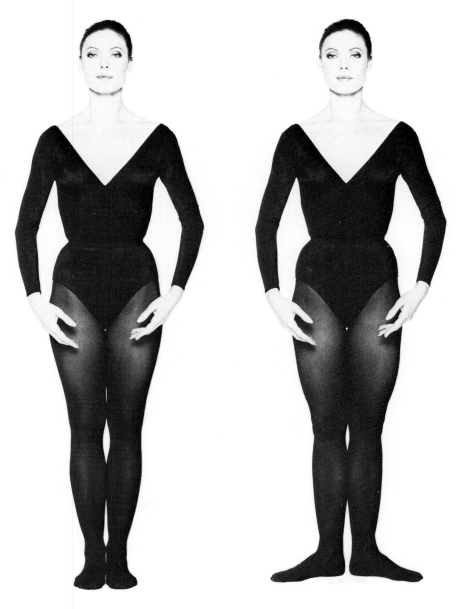

1. Stand up straight with your legs parallel, stomach in, buttocks pulled tight.

2. Then, slowly rotate both legs from the hip socket as far as you can with your knees still pointing over your toes. It doesn't matter if you can't turn your feet out as far as this, just do it as far as you can still keeping your knees over your toes. (If your knees are facing front, and your toes to the side, you can easily injure your knees.)

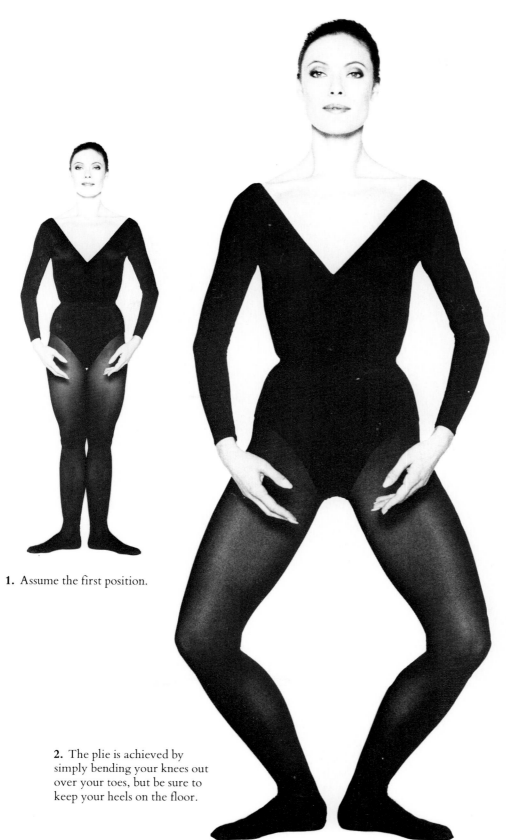

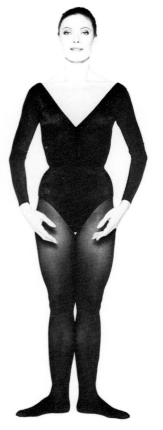

1. Assume the first position.

2. The plie is achieved by simply bending your knees out over your toes, but be sure to keep your heels on the floor.

3. Slowly straighten your knees, using resistance as though you're doing the exercise in water. Begin with 32 and work up to advanced, 64.

THE WORKOUT
4. Tendus

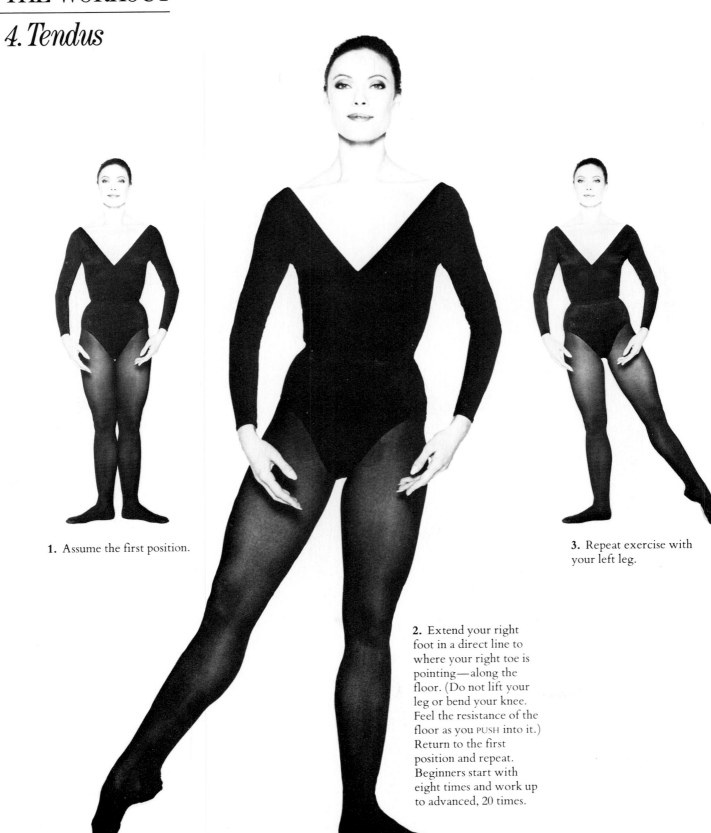

1. Assume the first position.

3. Repeat exercise with your left leg.

2. Extend your right foot in a direct line to where your right toe is pointing—along the floor. (Do not lift your leg or bend your knee. Feel the resistance of the floor as you PUSH into it.) Return to the first position and repeat. Beginners start with eight times and work up to advanced, 20 times.

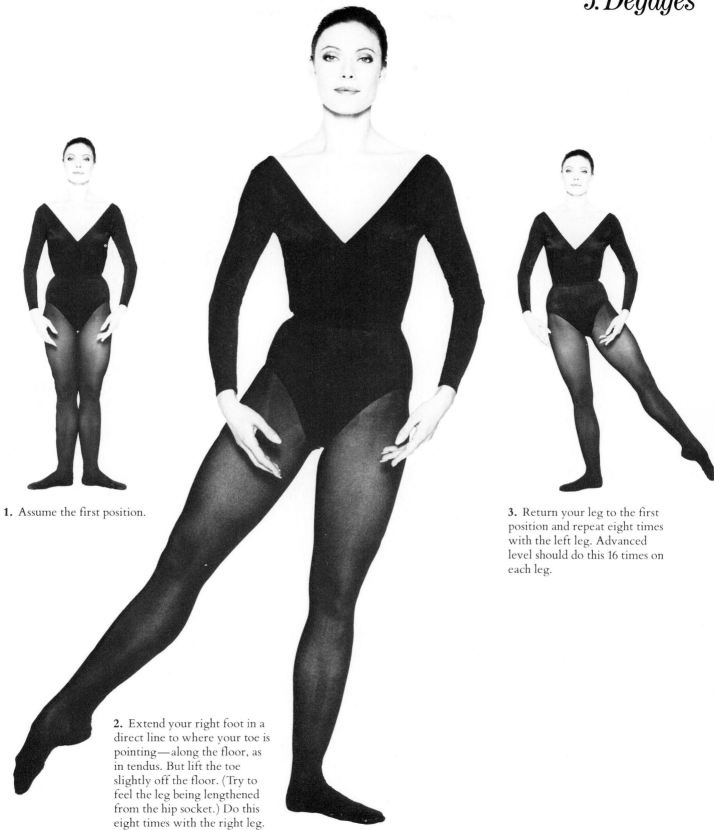

1. Assume the first position.

2. Extend your right foot in a direct line to where your toe is pointing—along the floor, as in tendus. But lift the toe slightly off the floor. (Try to feel the leg being lengthened from the hip socket.) Do this eight times with the right leg.

3. Return your leg to the first position and repeat eight times with the left leg. Advanced level should do this 16 times on each leg.

6. Relevés

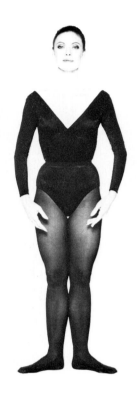

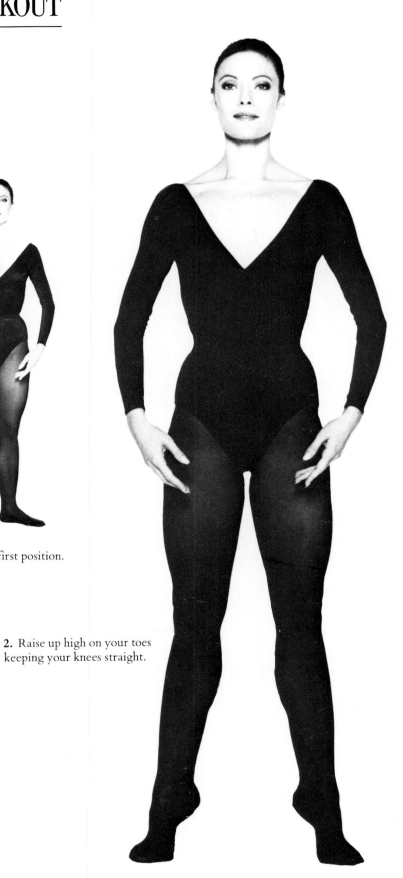

1. Assume the first position.

2. Raise up high on your toes keeping your knees straight.

3. Let your heels down and repeat. Begin with 32 times and work up to advanced, 64.

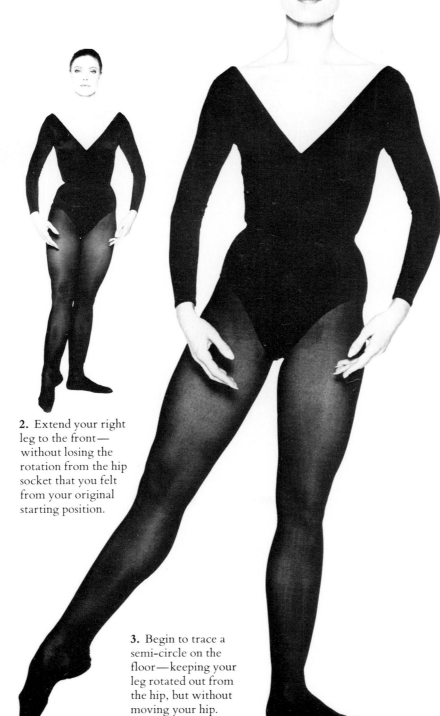
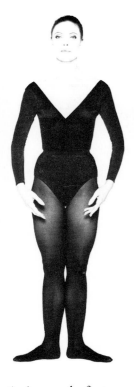

1. Assume the first position.

2. Extend your right leg to the front—without losing the rotation from the hip socket that you felt from your original starting position.

3. Begin to trace a semi-circle on the floor—keeping your leg rotated out from the hip, but without moving your hip.

4. Continue the semi-circle around until your leg is stretched out at the back. Do not let your knee bend or your hips move. Do not lose that outward rotation. Begin with eight circles on each leg and work up to 16 circles on each leg, advanced.

8. Doubled-Over Calf Raises

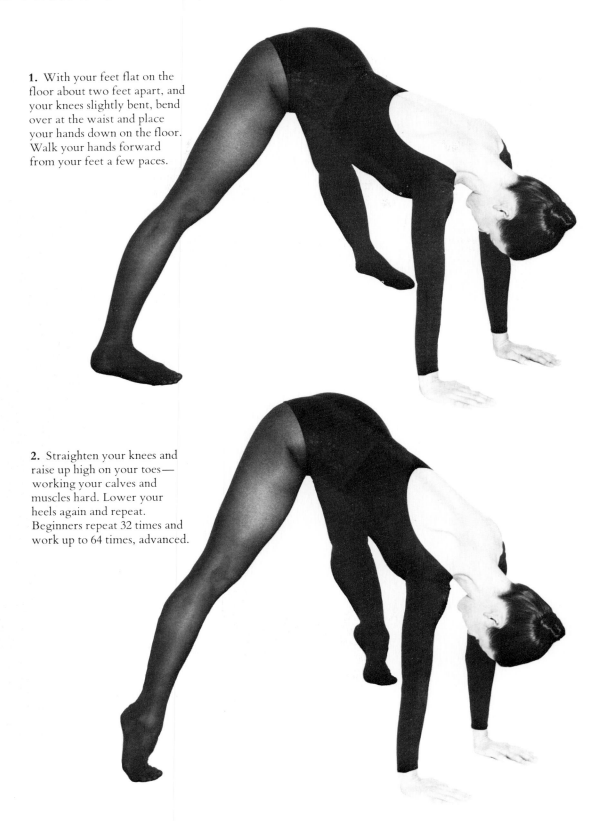

1. With your feet flat on the floor about two feet apart, and your knees slightly bent, bend over at the waist and place your hands down on the floor. Walk your hands forward from your feet a few paces.

2. Straighten your knees and raise up high on your toes — working your calves and muscles hard. Lower your heels again and repeat. Beginners repeat 32 times and work up to 64 times, advanced.

9. Thigh & Back Strengthener

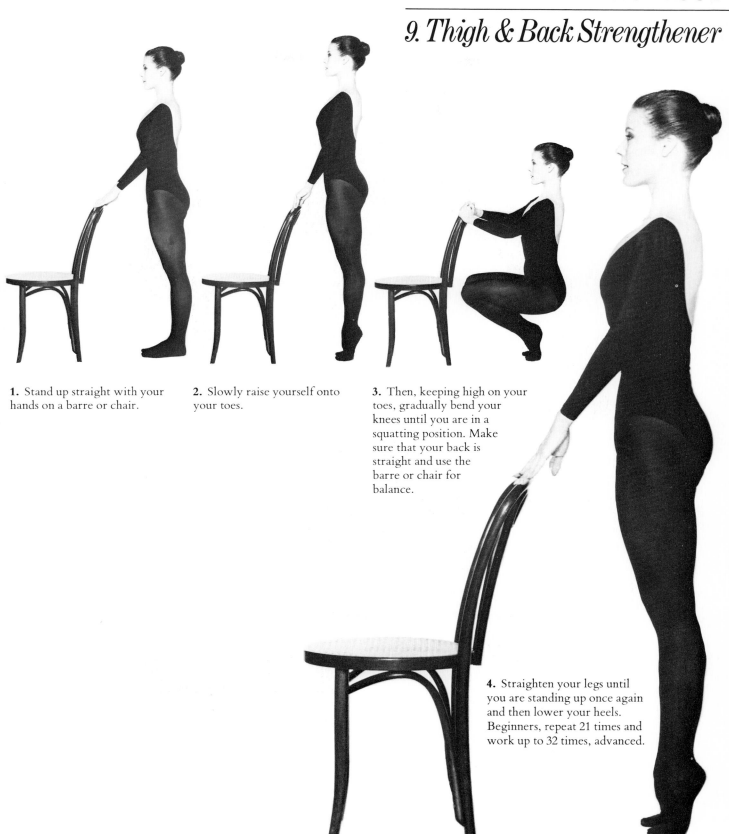

1. Stand up straight with your hands on a barre or chair.

2. Slowly raise yourself onto your toes.

3. Then, keeping high on your toes, gradually bend your knees until you are in a squatting position. Make sure that your back is straight and use the barre or chair for balance.

4. Straighten your legs until you are standing up once again and then lower your heels. Beginners, repeat 21 times and work up to 32 times, advanced.

10. Grand Battement

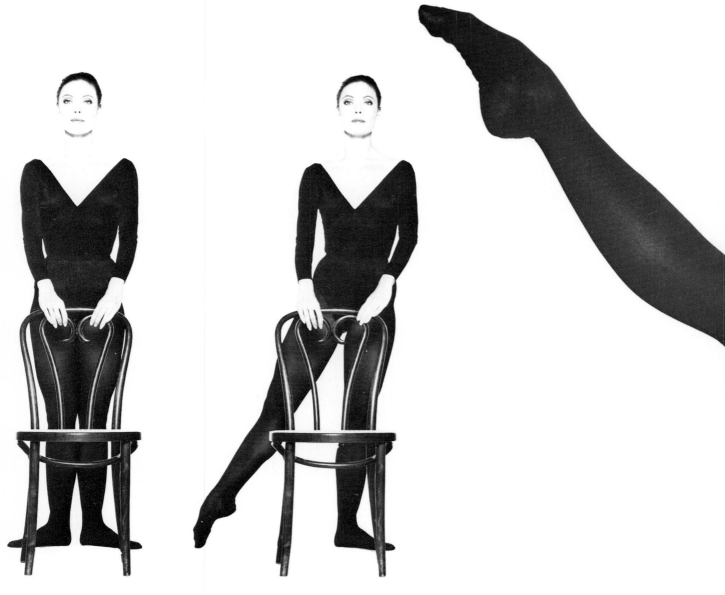

1. Assume the first position with hands on a barre or chair.

2. Extend your right foot out to the tendu position.

3. Lift your right leg to the side as high as you can without lifting your hip and trying to use your stomach muscles.

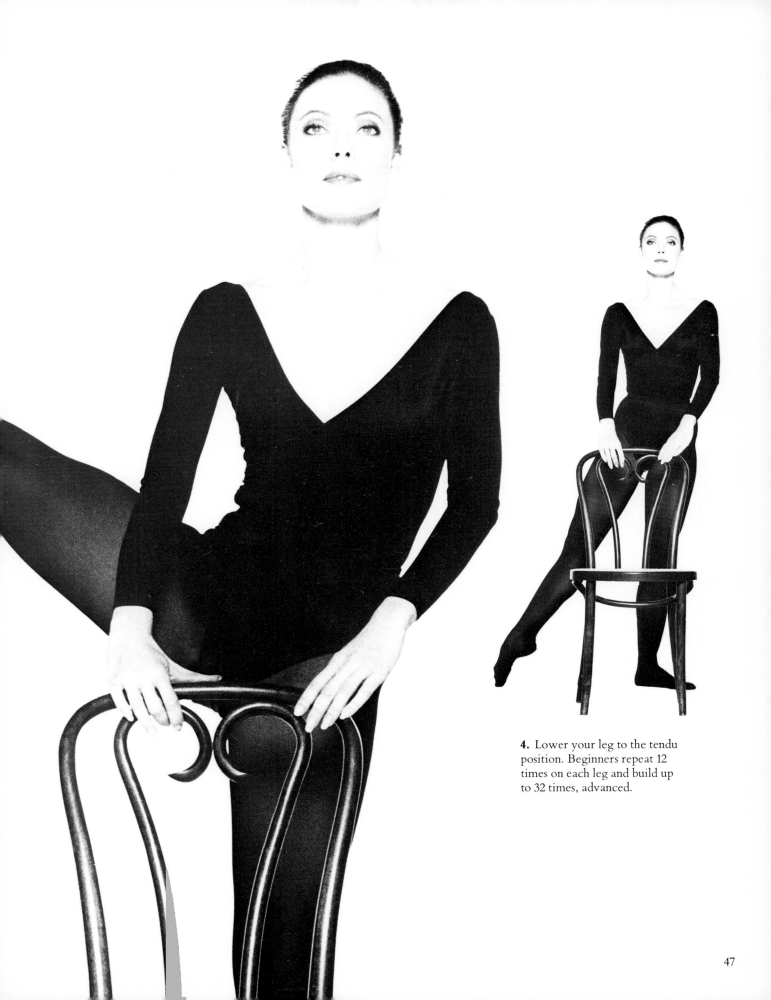

4. Lower your leg to the tendu position. Beginners repeat 12 times on each leg and build up to 32 times, advanced.

11. Battement Cloche

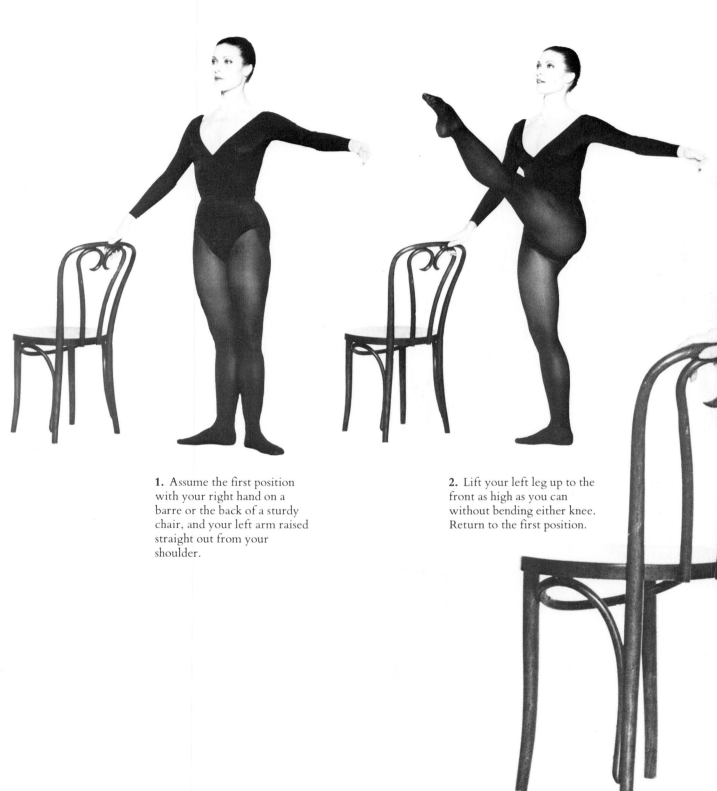

1. Assume the first position with your right hand on a barre or the back of a sturdy chair, and your left arm raised straight out from your shoulder.

2. Lift your left leg up to the front as high as you can without bending either knee. Return to the first position.

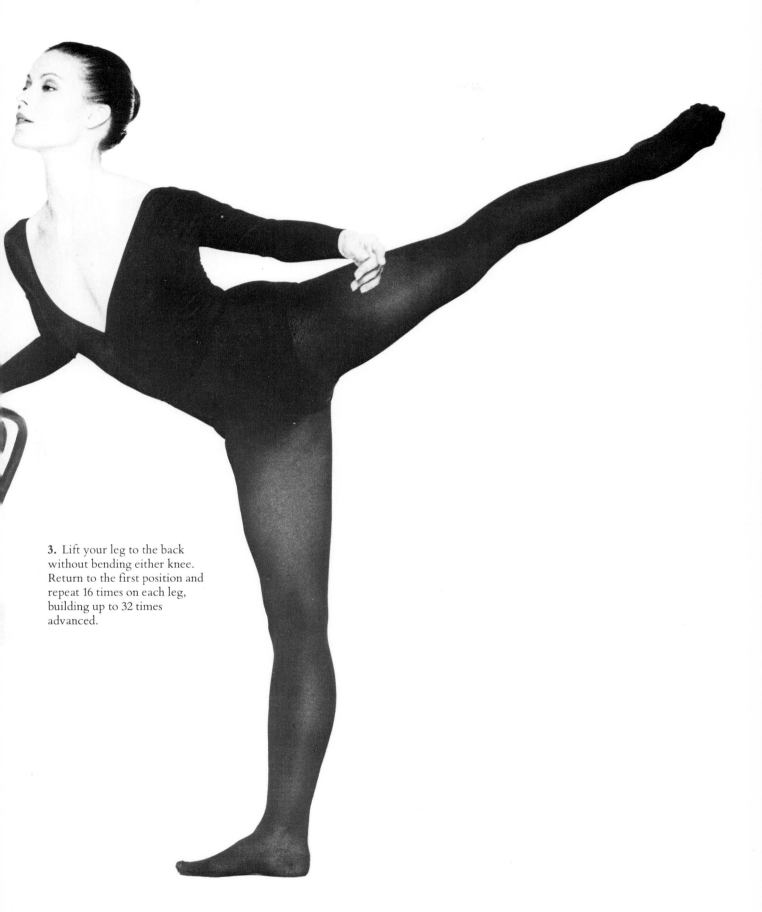

3. Lift your leg to the back
without bending either knee.
Return to the first position and
repeat 16 times on each leg,
building up to 32 times
advanced.

12. The Back-of-the-Leg Stretch

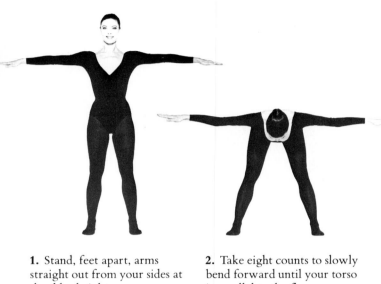

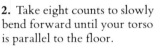

1. Stand, feet apart, arms straight out from your sides at shoulder height.

2. Take eight counts to slowly bend forward until your torso is parallel to the floor.

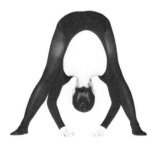

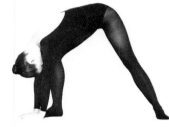

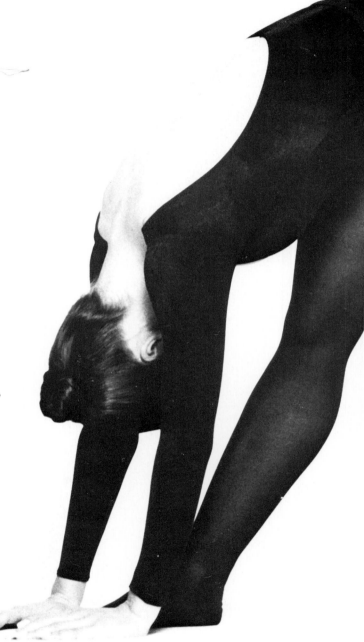

3. Now, continue dropping forward until your hands are relaxed on the floor. (Beginners may not be able to reach the floor and this may be painful when you start. But week by week you will notice that you will be able to go lower and lower.) Do this motion to the slow count of eight.

4. Walk your hands to your right foot. Try to put your chest on your right knee for eight counts.

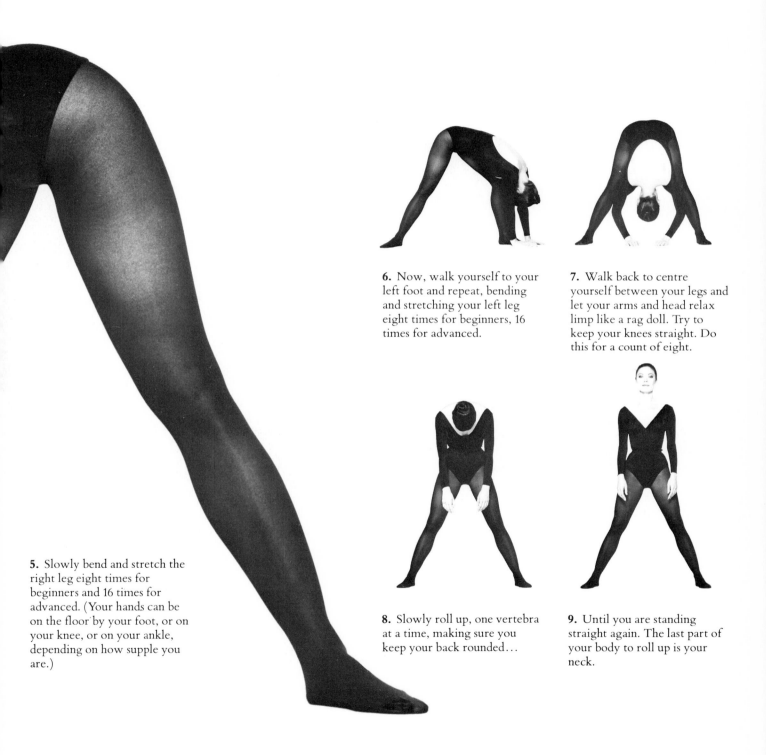

5. Slowly bend and stretch the right leg eight times for beginners and 16 times for advanced. (Your hands can be on the floor by your foot, or on your knee, or on your ankle, depending on how supple you are.)

6. Now, walk yourself to your left foot and repeat, bending and stretching your left leg eight times for beginners, 16 times for advanced.

7. Walk back to centre yourself between your legs and let your arms and head relax limp like a rag doll. Try to keep your knees straight. Do this for a count of eight.

8. Slowly roll up, one vertebra at a time, making sure you keep your back rounded...

9. Until you are standing straight again. The last part of your body to roll up is your neck.

THE WORKOUT

13. Partial Sit-Ups

Please read the chapter on posture and make sure you understand the *Pelvic Tilt* before attempting any of the following three exercises.

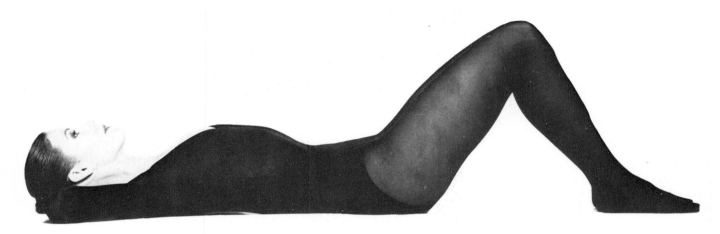

1. Lie on the floor, your hands behind your neck, elbows back. Bend your knees and keep your feet apart in line with your hip bones.

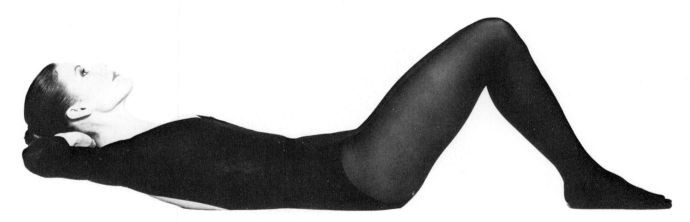

2. Pull in your stomach muscles and use them to lift your head and upper back only off the floor. (Make sure you are flattening your stomach muscles as you use them, and don't let them bunch out. And don't cheat by letting your elbows come forward to help lift yourself. If you think you're cheating, stop, rest, and then begin again.) Using your stomach muscles, lower your back toward the floor—but not quite touching it. Repeat the movement 24 times for beginners and 64 times for advanced.

1. Lie on the floor, knees bent, feet in line with your hip bones, arms relaxed at your sides.

2. Using your stomach muscles, lift your upper body off the floor and reach your arms forward through your knees.

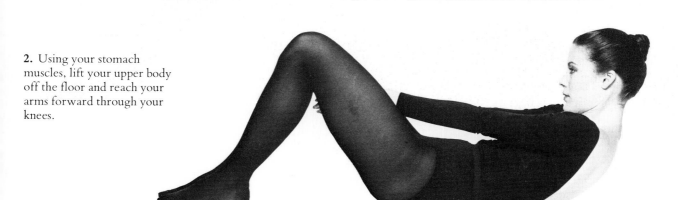

3. Now, reach with your right arm as far as you can through your knees.

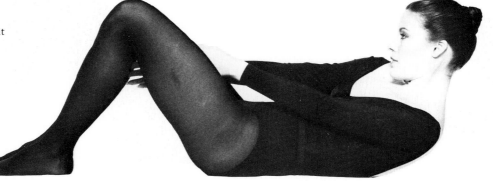

4. Then, reach your left arm as far as you can, allowing your right arm to come back slightly. Repeat 32 times for beginners and 64 times for advanced. When you are finished, roll slowly back to the starting position, keeping your back rounded and letting yourself down vertebra by vertebra.

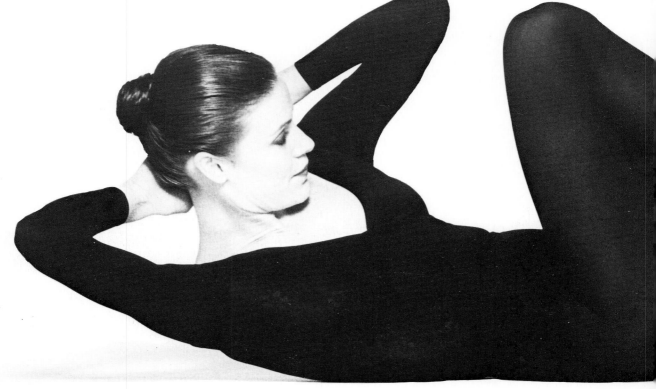

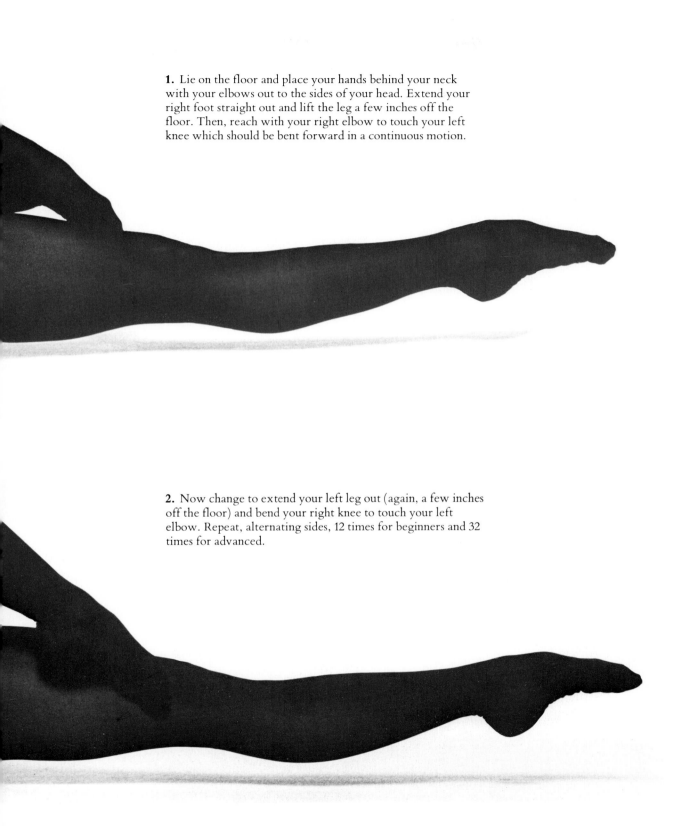

1. Lie on the floor and place your hands behind your neck with your elbows out to the sides of your head. Extend your right foot straight out and lift the leg a few inches off the floor. Then, reach with your right elbow to touch your left knee which should be bent forward in a continuous motion.

2. Now change to extend your left leg out (again, a few inches off the floor) and bend your right knee to touch your left elbow. Repeat, alternating sides, 12 times for beginners and 32 times for advanced.

THE WORKOUT
16. Side Leg Lifts

1. Lie on your left side, putting your upper body weight on your left elbow, both palms flat on the floor. Stretch your legs—the top parallel to the bottom.

2. With your toes pointed, lift your right leg up. Keeping your legs parallel, you should not be able to lift your leg higher than this, if you're doing it correctly.

3. Lower your right leg, with resistance, to within a few inches of your bottom leg. Repeat 24 times for beginners with the foot pointed, and then 24 times with the foot flexed. Then change legs and repeat. Advanced do both legs 48 times. (When you are finished with each leg you should grab your ankle and stretch your thigh muscles.)

17. Tricky Crossovers

1. Lie on your left side, your upper torso up on your left elbow, palms flat on the floor. (Don't sink into your left elbow; hold yourself up!) Extend your left leg straight down in line with your upper body but bend it at the knee. When you cross over your right leg, keep it straight.

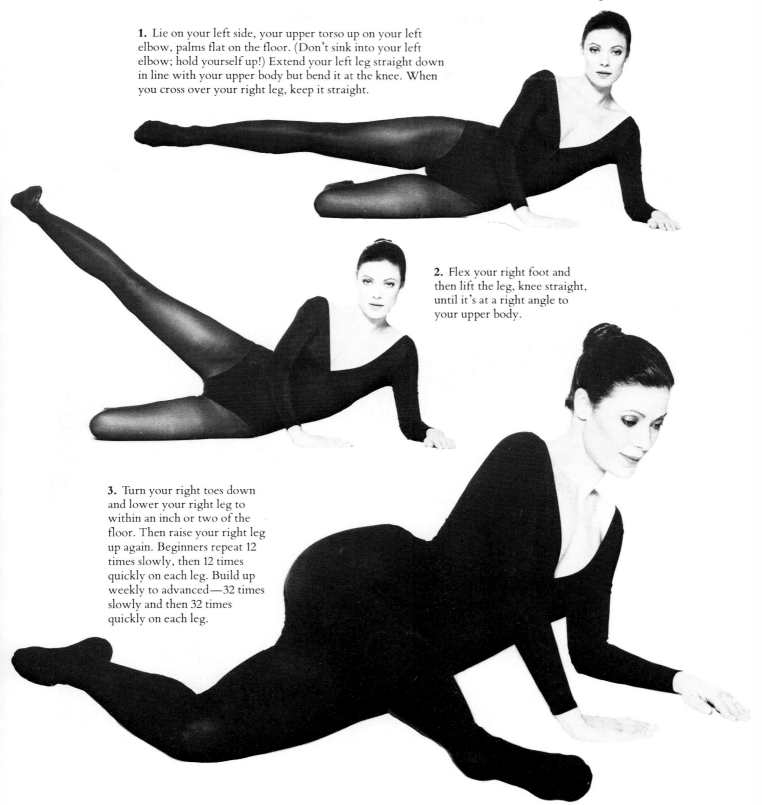

2. Flex your right foot and then lift the leg, knee straight, until it's at a right angle to your upper body.

3. Turn your right toes down and lower your right leg to within an inch or two of the floor. Then raise your right leg up again. Beginners repeat 12 times slowly, then 12 times quickly on each leg. Build up weekly to advanced—32 times slowly and then 32 times quickly on each leg.

57

THE WORKOUT

19. The Scissor Kick

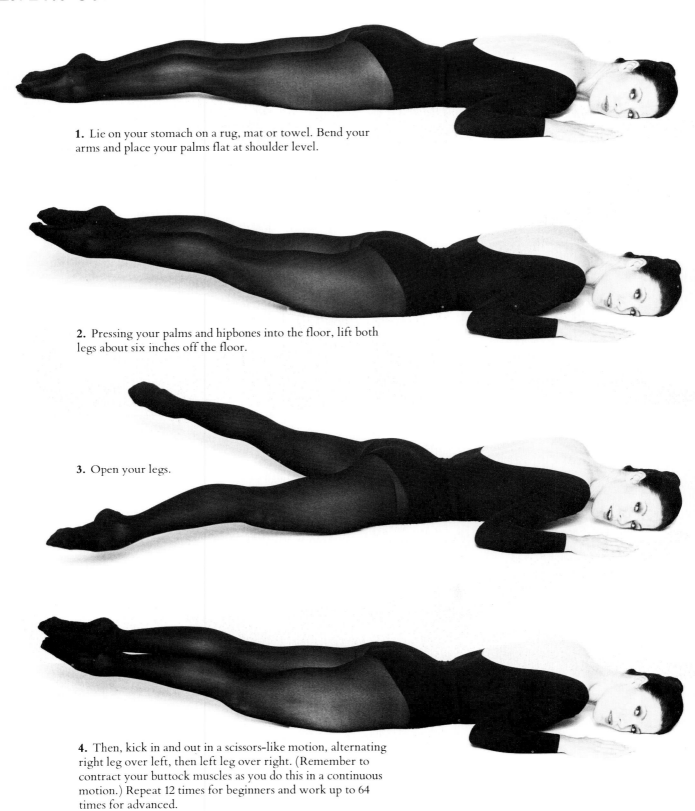

1. Lie on your stomach on a rug, mat or towel. Bend your arms and place your palms flat at shoulder level.

2. Pressing your palms and hipbones into the floor, lift both legs about six inches off the floor.

3. Open your legs.

4. Then, kick in and out in a scissors-like motion, alternating right leg over left, then left leg over right. (Remember to contract your buttock muscles as you do this in a continuous motion.) Repeat 12 times for beginners and work up to 64 times for advanced.

20. Rear Leg Raises

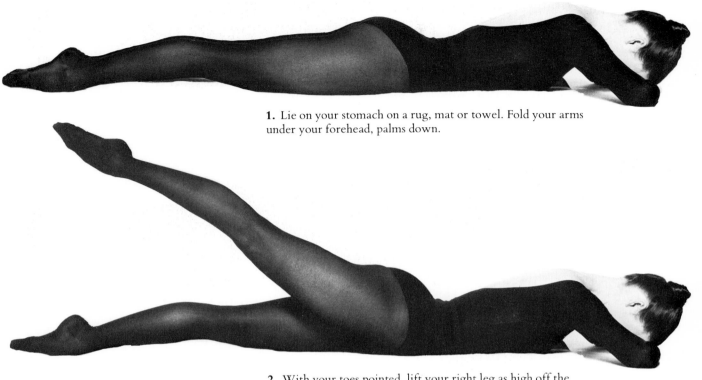

1. Lie on your stomach on a rug, mat or towel. Fold your arms under your forehead, palms down.

2. With your toes pointed, lift your right leg as high off the floor as it will go without lifting your hipbones off the floor and keeping your legs straight.

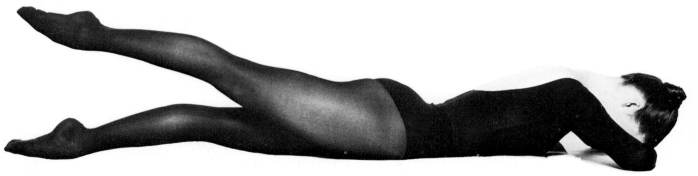

3. Now, lower your right leg about one foot and then raise it again. Continue this movement up and down, 12 times on each leg for beginners and 32 times each leg for advanced.

21. Arched Kicks

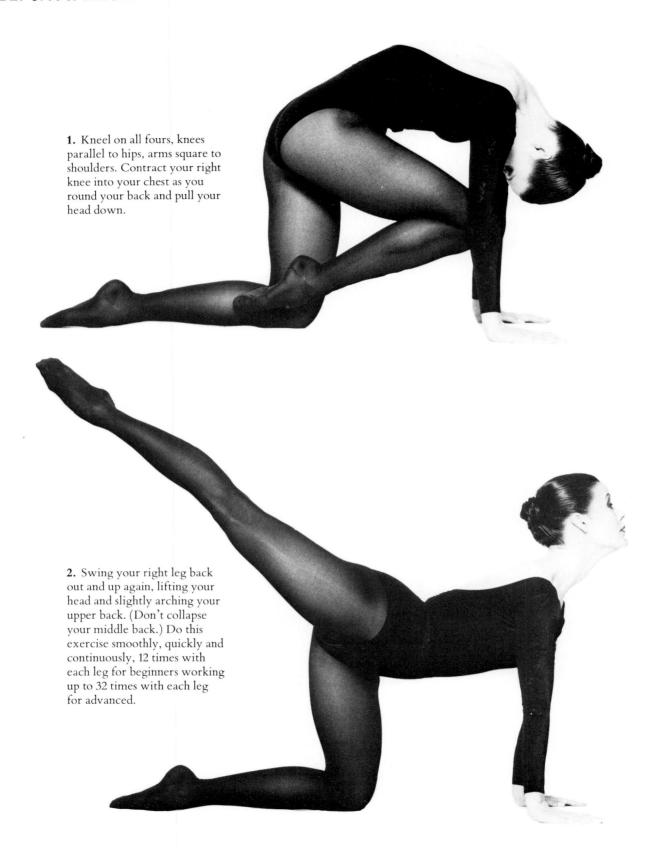

1. Kneel on all fours, knees parallel to hips, arms square to shoulders. Contract your right knee into your chest as you round your back and pull your head down.

2. Swing your right leg back out and up again, lifting your head and slightly arching your upper back. (Don't collapse your middle back.) Do this exercise smoothly, quickly and continuously, 12 times with each leg for beginners working up to 32 times with each leg for advanced.

22. Back Leg Extensions

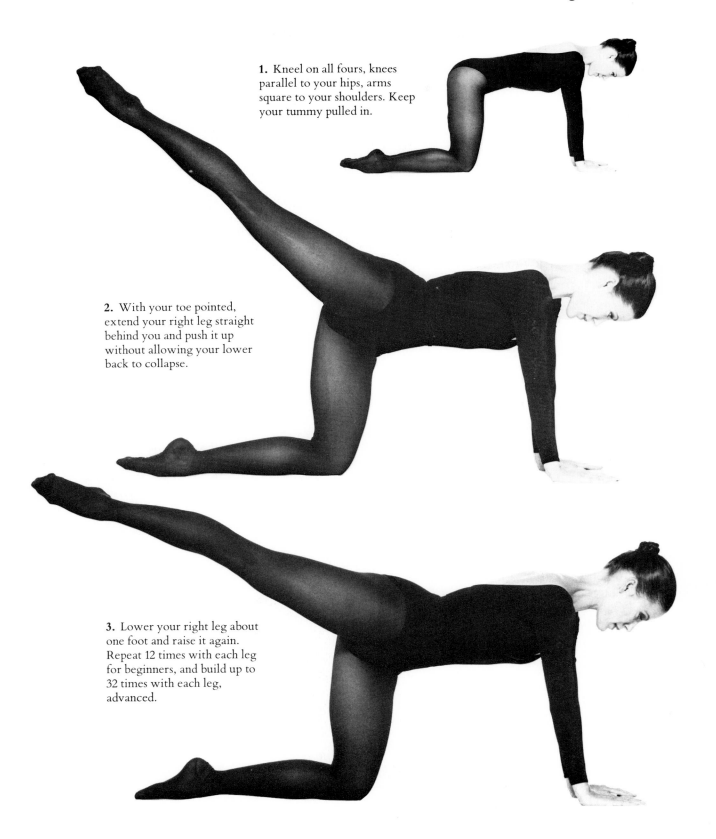

1. Kneel on all fours, knees parallel to your hips, arms square to your shoulders. Keep your tummy pulled in.

2. With your toe pointed, extend your right leg straight behind you and push it up without allowing your lower back to collapse.

3. Lower your right leg about one foot and raise it again. Repeat 12 times with each leg for beginners, and build up to 32 times with each leg, advanced.

23. Front Thigh Stretch

1. Lie on your left side, up on your left elbow, with your left palm flat on the floor. Extend your left leg straight out on a line with your upper body, but bend your right leg at the knee. Grab your right foot with your right hand and stretch your foot into your buttocks.

2. Roll over onto your back so that your right leg is bent under your body. Lie this way for the count of 10. Repeat with your other leg.

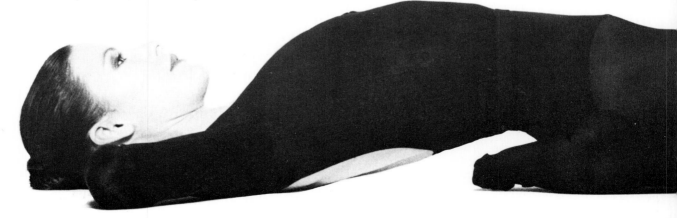

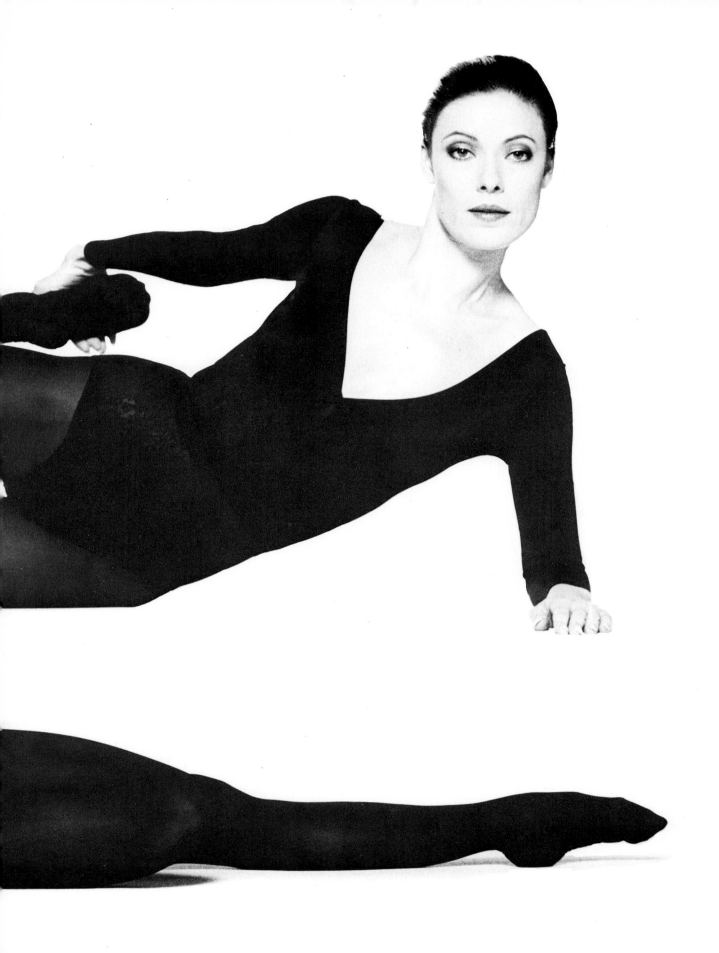

THE WORKOUT
24. The Elbow Side Stretch

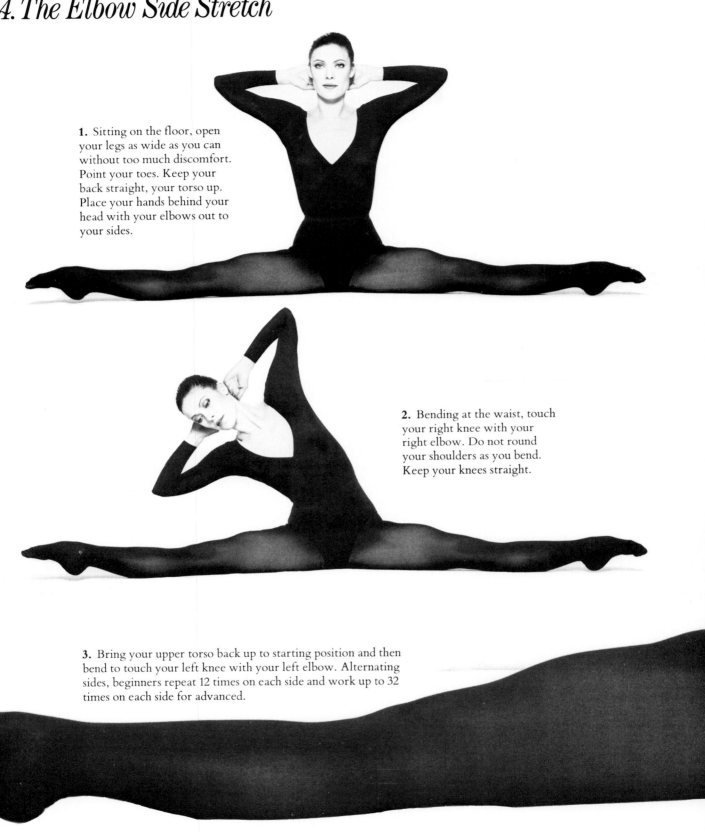

1. Sitting on the floor, open your legs as wide as you can without too much discomfort. Point your toes. Keep your back straight, your torso up. Place your hands behind your head with your elbows out to your sides.

2. Bending at the waist, touch your right knee with your right elbow. Do not round your shoulders as you bend. Keep your knees straight.

3. Bring your upper torso back up to starting position and then bend to touch your left knee with your left elbow. Alternating sides, beginners repeat 12 times on each side and work up to 32 times on each side for advanced.

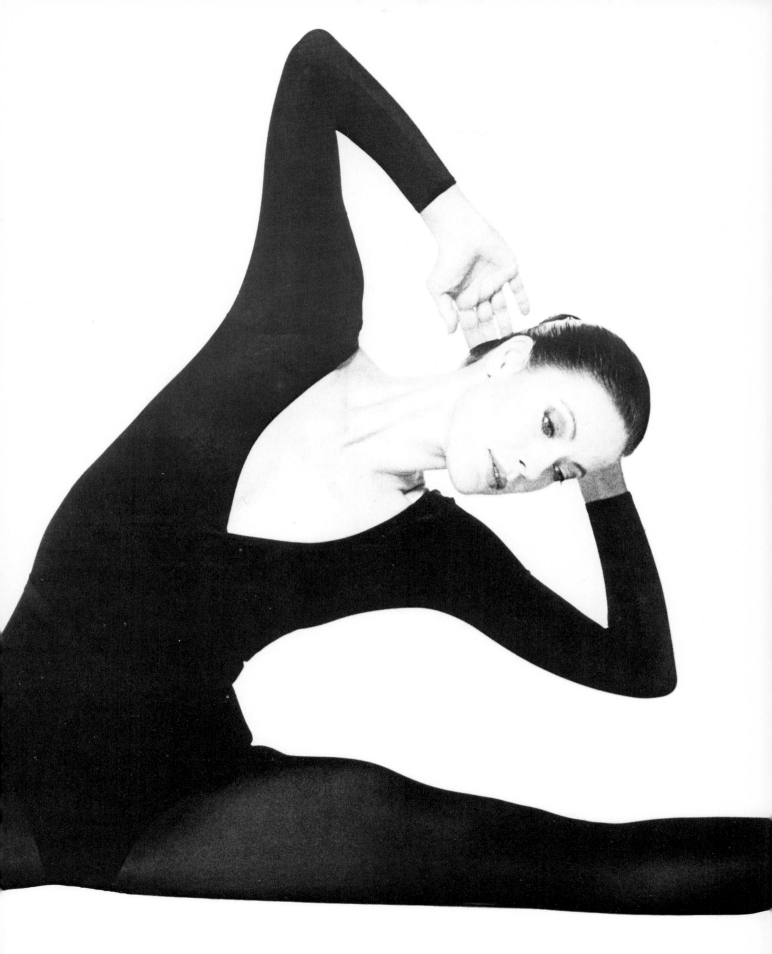

25. The Killer Stretch

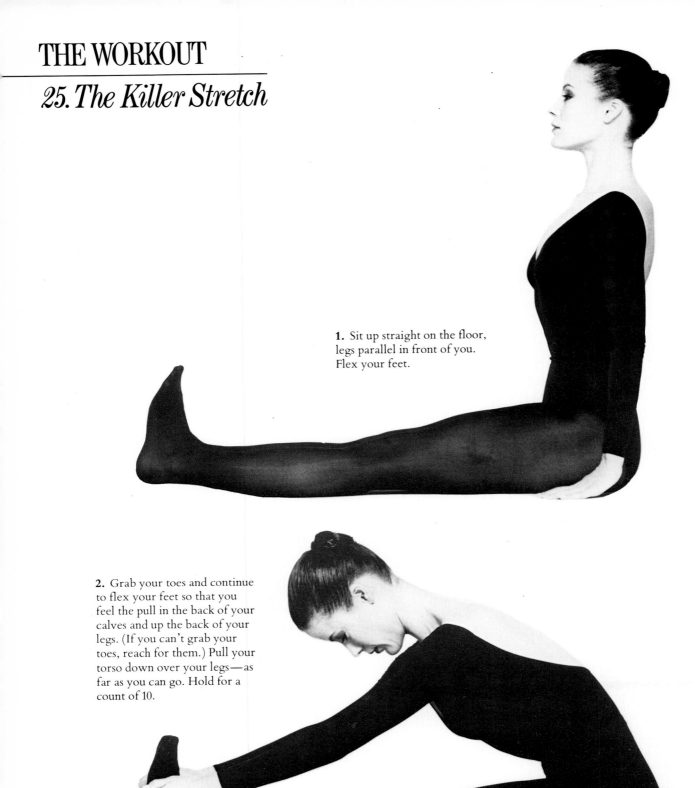

1. Sit up straight on the floor, legs parallel in front of you. Flex your feet.

2. Grab your toes and continue to flex your feet so that you feel the pull in the back of your calves and up the back of your legs. (If you can't grab your toes, reach for them.) Pull your torso down over your legs—as far as you can go. Hold for a count of 10.

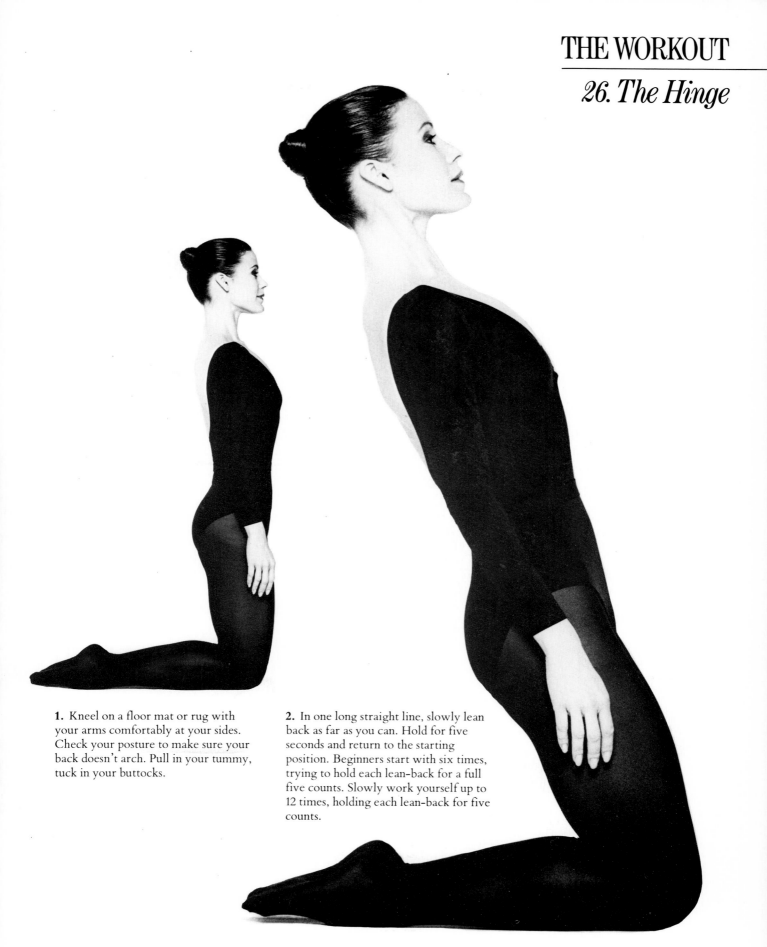

1. Kneel on a floor mat or rug with your arms comfortably at your sides. Check your posture to make sure your back doesn't arch. Pull in your tummy, tuck in your buttocks.

2. In one long straight line, slowly lean back as far as you can. Hold for five seconds and return to the starting position. Beginners start with six times, trying to hold each lean-back for a full five counts. Slowly work yourself up to 12 times, holding each lean-back for five counts.

THE WORKOUT

27. Buttocks Lifts

1. Lie flat on your back, knees bent, feet parallel about hip distance apart. Rest your arms alongside your body.

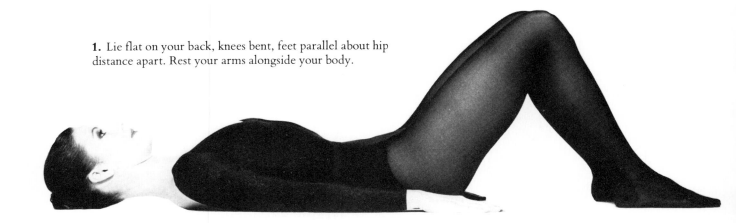

2. With your knees and feet parallel, shift your weight onto your shoulders and lift your buttocks—squeezing as hard as you can. Then, keeping your hips high, relax those muscles slightly. (Your hips may drop an inch or two.) Repeat this contracting and relaxing of your buttocks muscles 32 times for beginners and work up to 64 times, advanced.

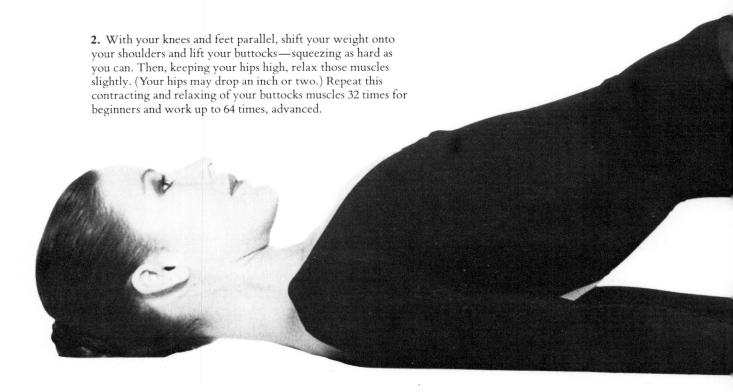

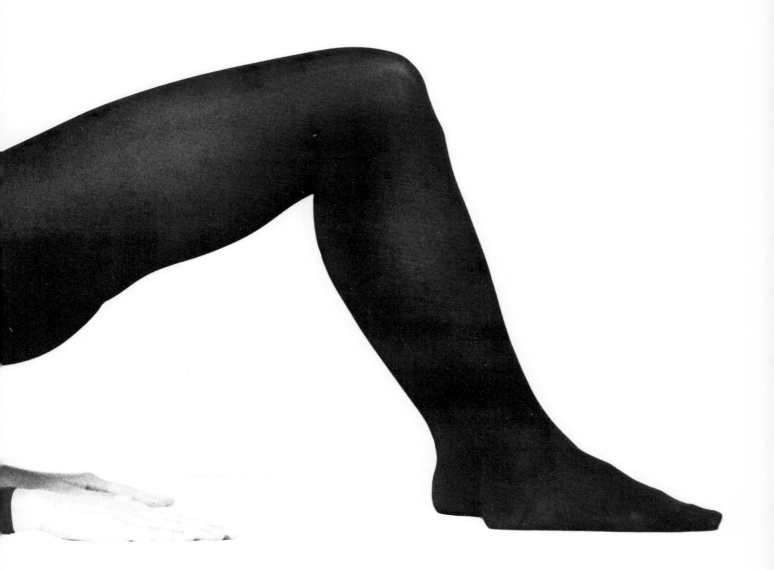

THE WORKOUT

28. Side Leg Extensions

1. Kneel on all fours, knees parallel to hips, arms square to your shoulders. Keep your back flat, your tummy pulled in, your head up.

2. Lift your right knee out to the side so that your knee is bent and lifted to hip height and your thigh is parallel to the floor and perpendicular to your hip.

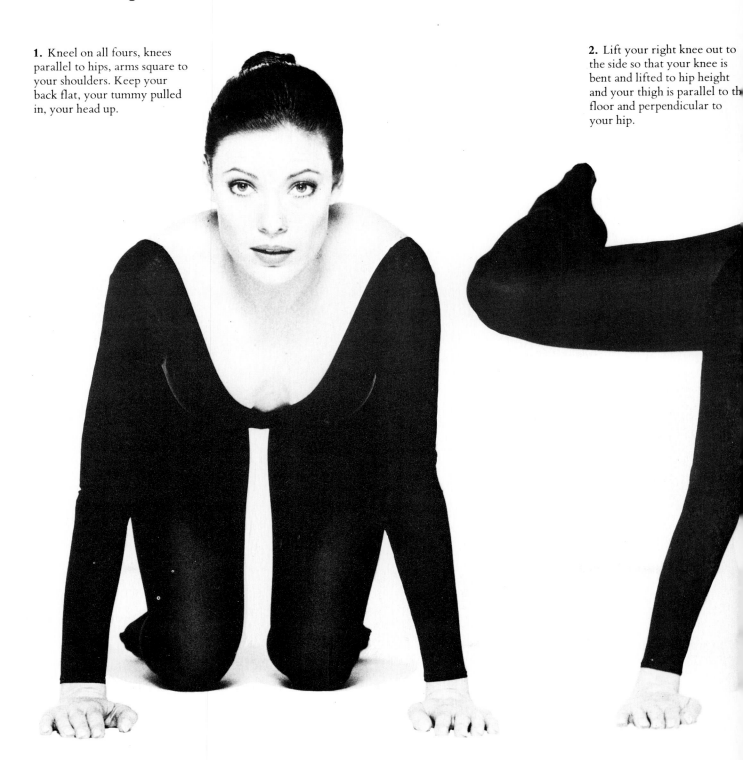

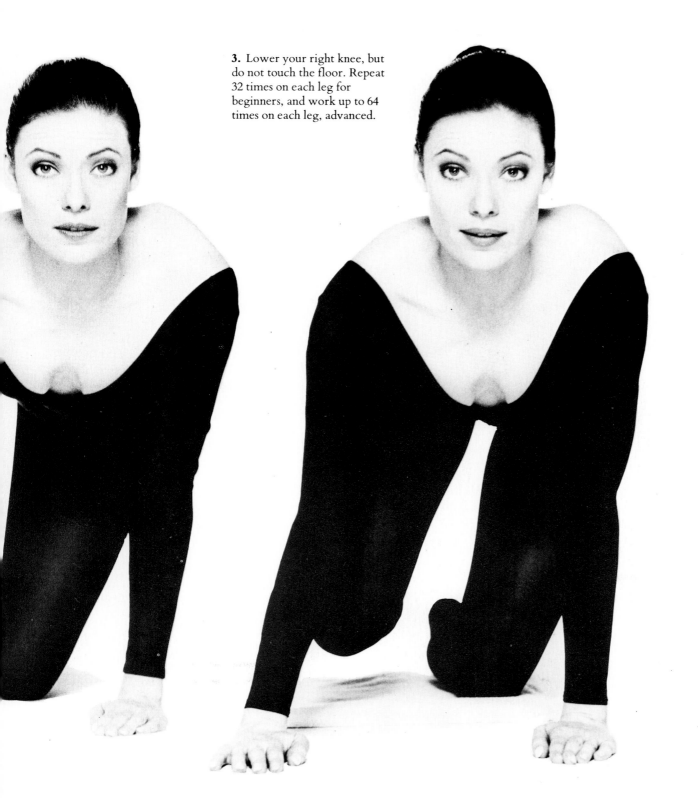

3. Lower your right knee, but do not touch the floor. Repeat 32 times on each leg for beginners, and work up to 64 times on each leg, advanced.

THE WORKOUT

29. Around the World

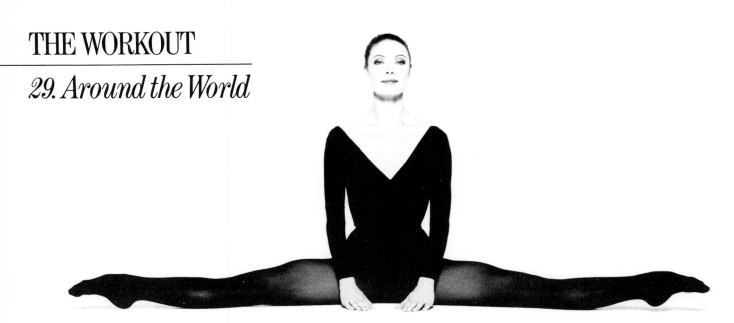

1. Sitting on the floor, open your legs as wide as you can without too much discomfort. Point your toes.

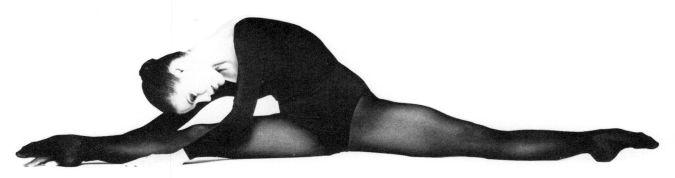

2. Slowly walk your hands down to your right leg. Let your body weight help you to relax into the stretch. Try to pull your chest onto your knee.

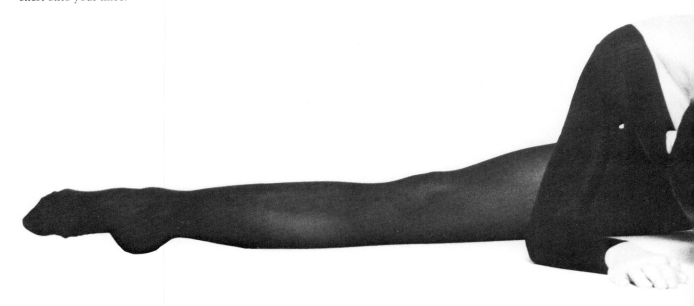

5. Now, from the sitting position, slowly walk your hands to the centre again and let your body weight pull you down far

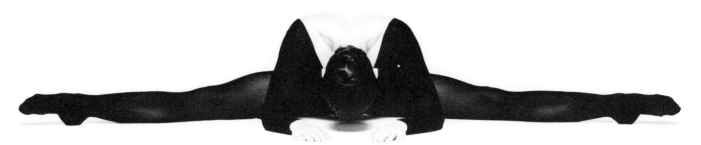

3. With your hands on the floor in front of you, slowly stretch out from your hip and walk yourself around to the front—keeping your chest and torso as low as you can to the floor.

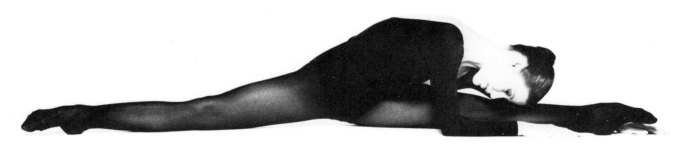

4. Then walk slowly to the left side. Again, try to pull your chest onto your knee. Straighten up to starting position, sitting up. Go round again, four times to the right and four times to the left.

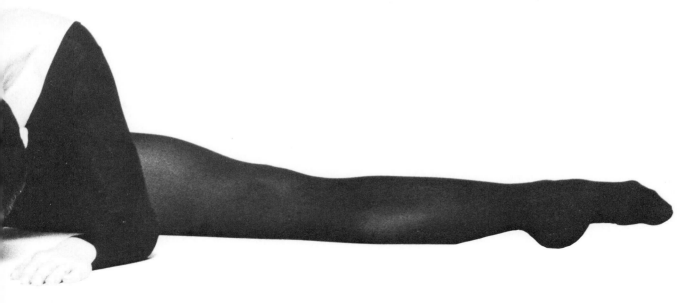

farther into the stretch. (The more you relax, the easier it is.) Advanced can also try this exercise with the feet flexed.

THE WORKOUT

30. *Just a Stretch*

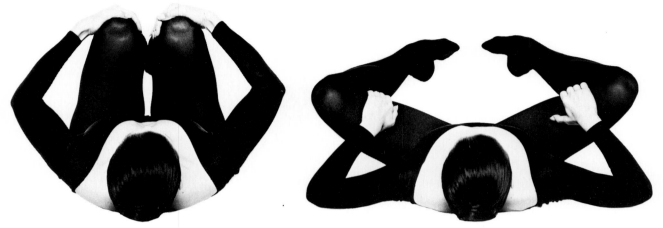

1. Lie flat on your back and bend both your knees into your torso—pulling them towards yourself with your hands holding your legs just below the knees. Don't let your back leave the floor.

2. Open your knees out to the sides. Place your hands on the insides of your thighs just above your knees and press down towards the floor, releasing slightly between presses, for the count of 16.

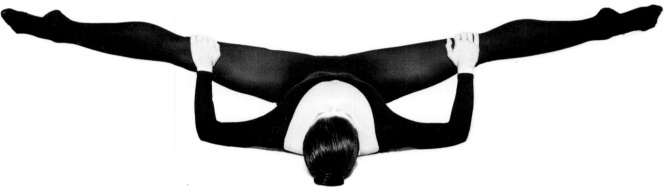

3. Holding your knees where you are, extend the lower part of your legs. Open your legs as wide as you can, stretching your feet straight out, to the slow count of 16. Still holding your knees where they are, bend the lower legs back to picture 2. Then hug your knees to your chest as in the starting position.

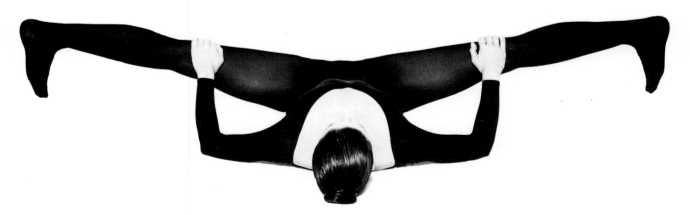

4. If you're up to it, flex your feet in the open position for a greater stretch. Beginners repeat this exercise four times and work up to 12 times, advanced.

The Wind-Down

THE WIND-DOWN

1. The Plough

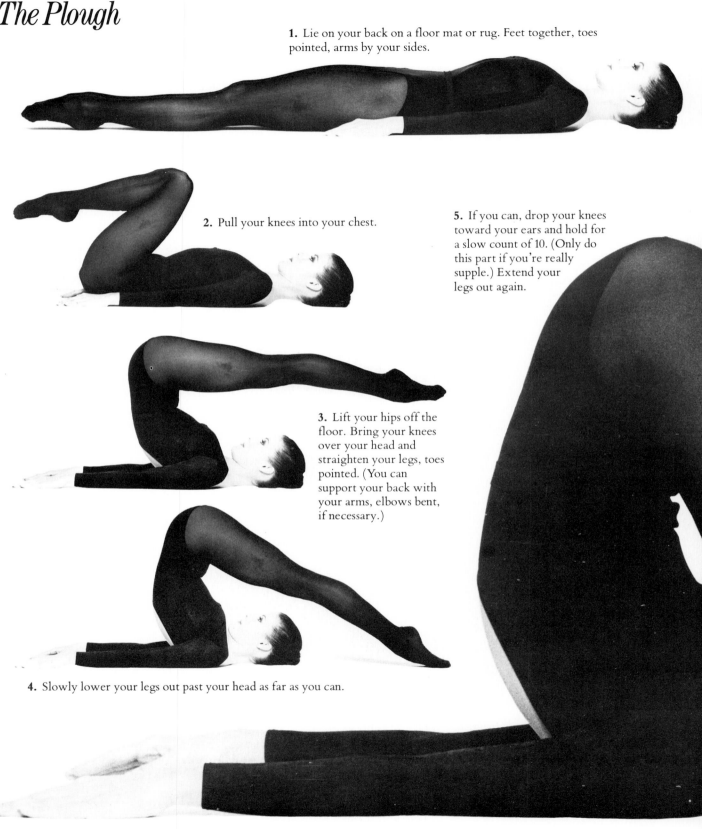

1. Lie on your back on a floor mat or rug. Feet together, toes pointed, arms by your sides.

2. Pull your knees into your chest.

5. If you can, drop your knees toward your ears and hold for a slow count of 10. (Only do this part if you're really supple.) Extend your legs out again.

3. Lift your hips off the floor. Bring your knees over your head and straighten your legs, toes pointed. (You can support your back with your arms, elbows bent, if necessary.)

4. Slowly lower your legs out past your head as far as you can.

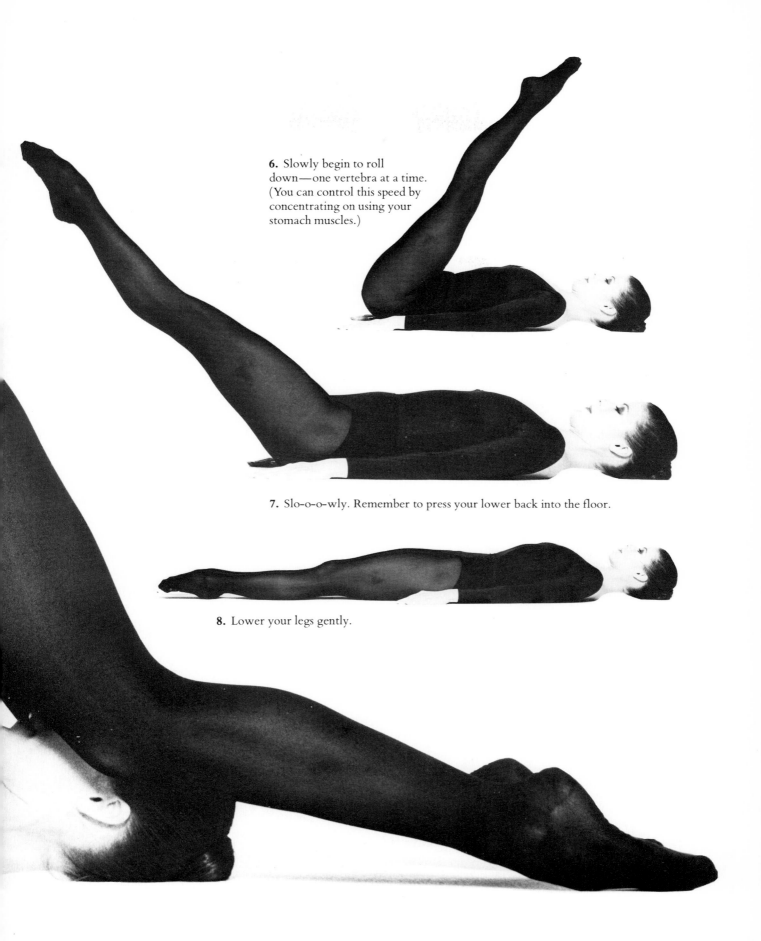

6. Slowly begin to roll down—one vertebra at a time. (You can control this speed by concentrating on using your stomach muscles.)

7. Slo-o-o-wly. Remember to press your lower back into the floor.

8. Lower your legs gently.

THE WIND-DOWN
2. Praying Stretch

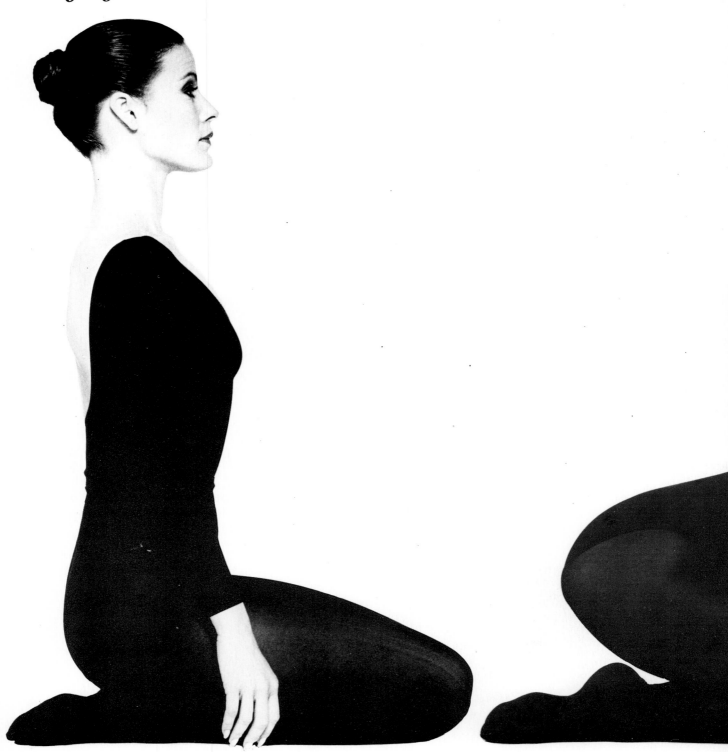

1. Kneel on a floor mat or rug and sit back on your heels.
Keep your back straight and your arms by your sides.

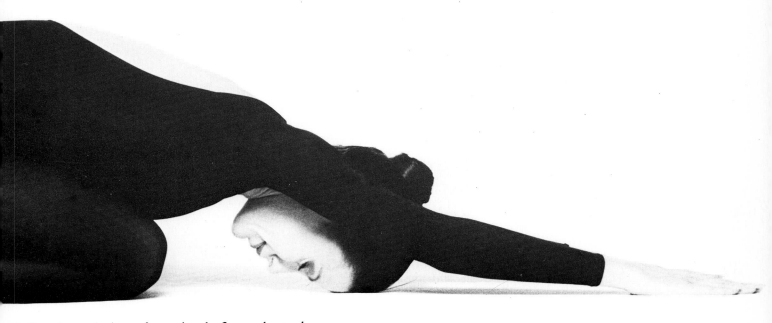

2. Stretch your body out forward to the floor and extend your
arms out as far in front as you can. Keep your head down.
Hold this position for as long as you want.

THE WIND-DOWN
3. Topsy Turvy

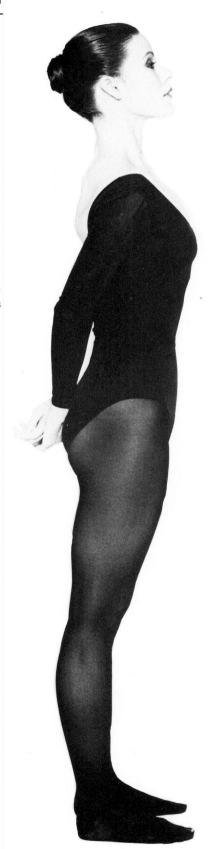

1. Stand with your feet about one foot apart and your hands clasped behind your back.

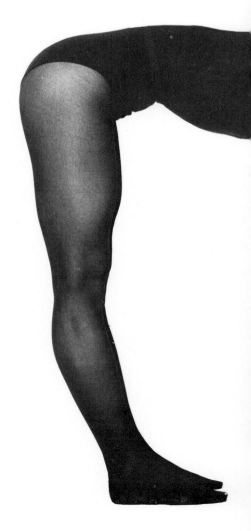

2. Keeping your hands clasped behind your back, begin to bend forward, slowly.

3. As you drop your head closer towards your knees, let your arms (still clasped) fall as far over your head as you can, stretching out your shoulders. Hold for a count of 10.

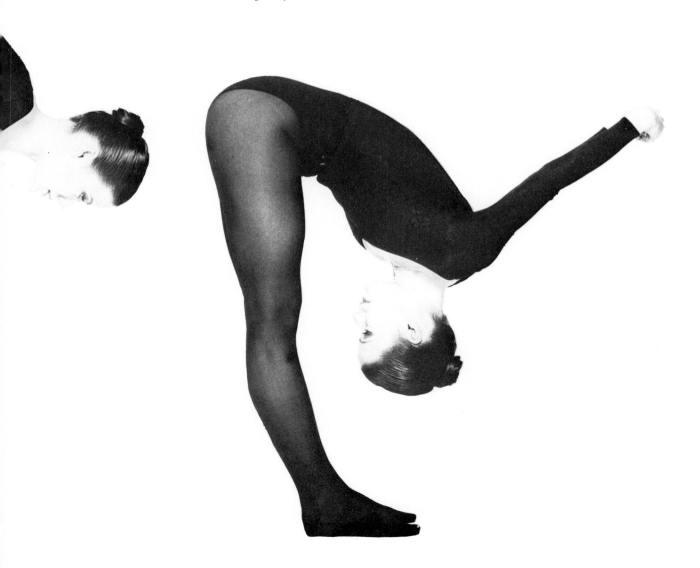

THE WIND-DOWN
4. Nose-to-Toes Stretch

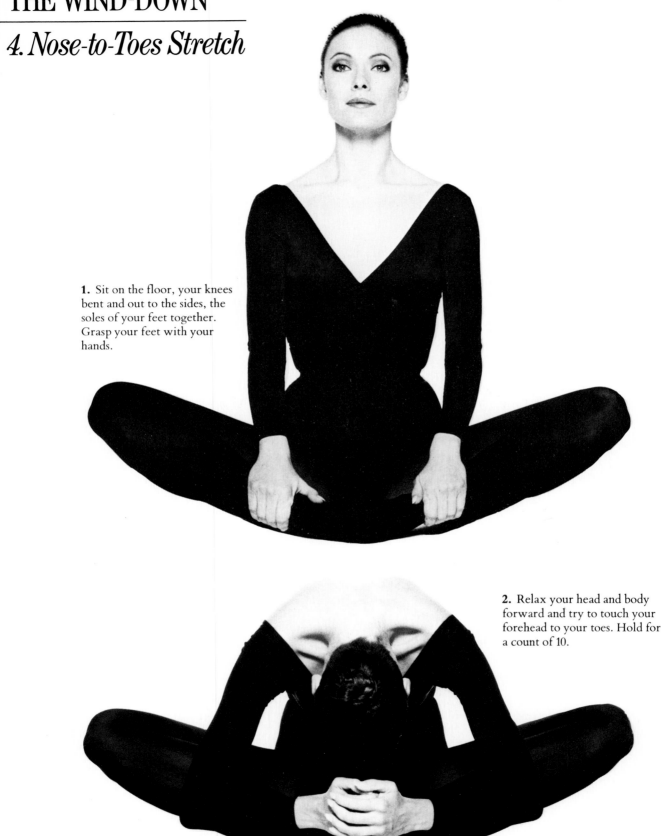

1. Sit on the floor, your knees bent and out to the sides, the soles of your feet together. Grasp your feet with your hands.

2. Relax your head and body forward and try to touch your forehead to your toes. Hold for a count of 10.

The Tough-it-Out Seven

THE TOUGH-IT-OUT SEVEN

1. The Incline

1. Lie on the floor, legs together, arms at your sides with the palms down, knees bent.

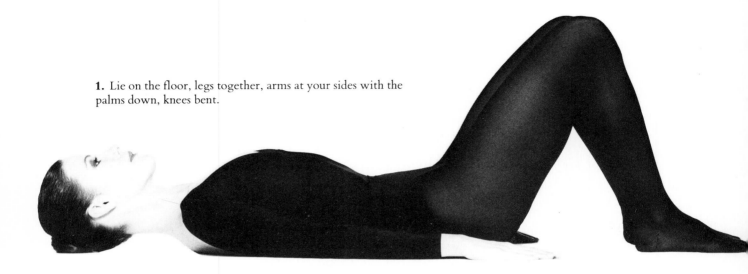

2. Squeeze in your buttocks and raise your hips off the floor. Extend your left leg straight out, toe pointed. Then, lower your hips and leg to the starting position and repeat with the right leg. Do 10 of these on each leg.

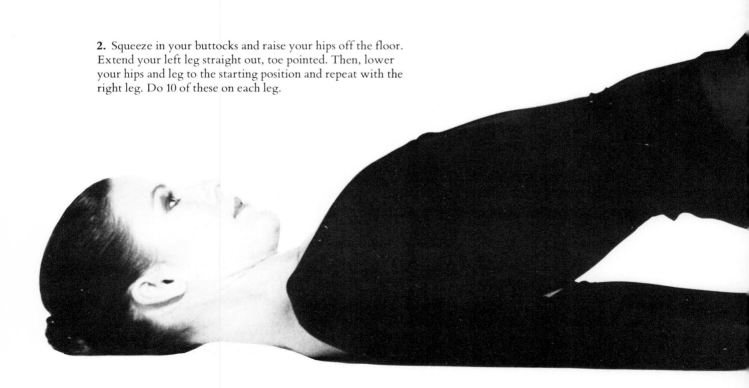

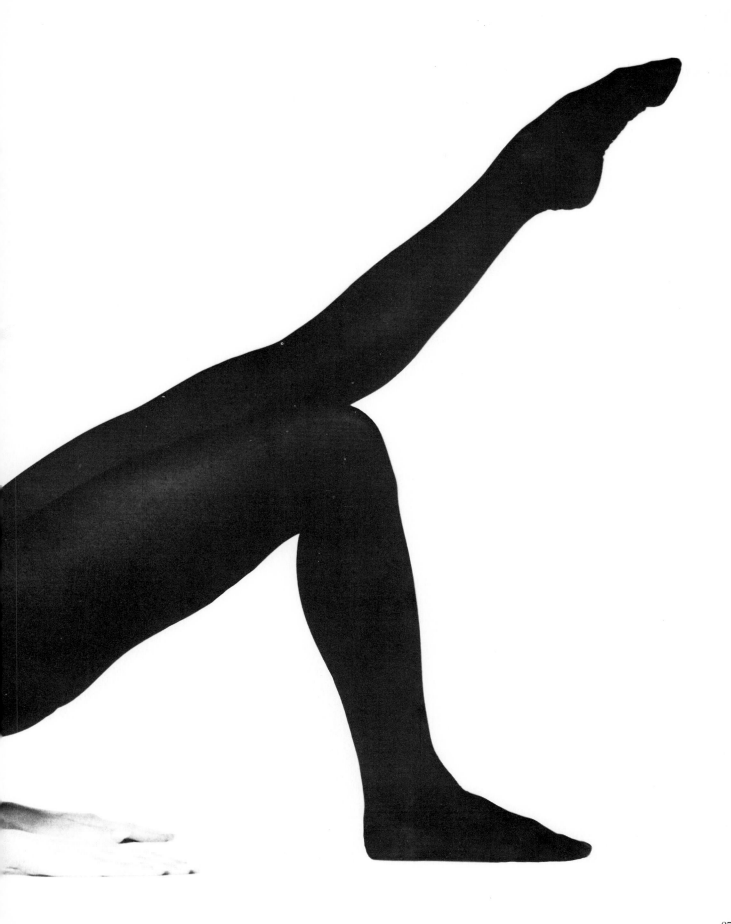

2. Extended Scissor Kicks

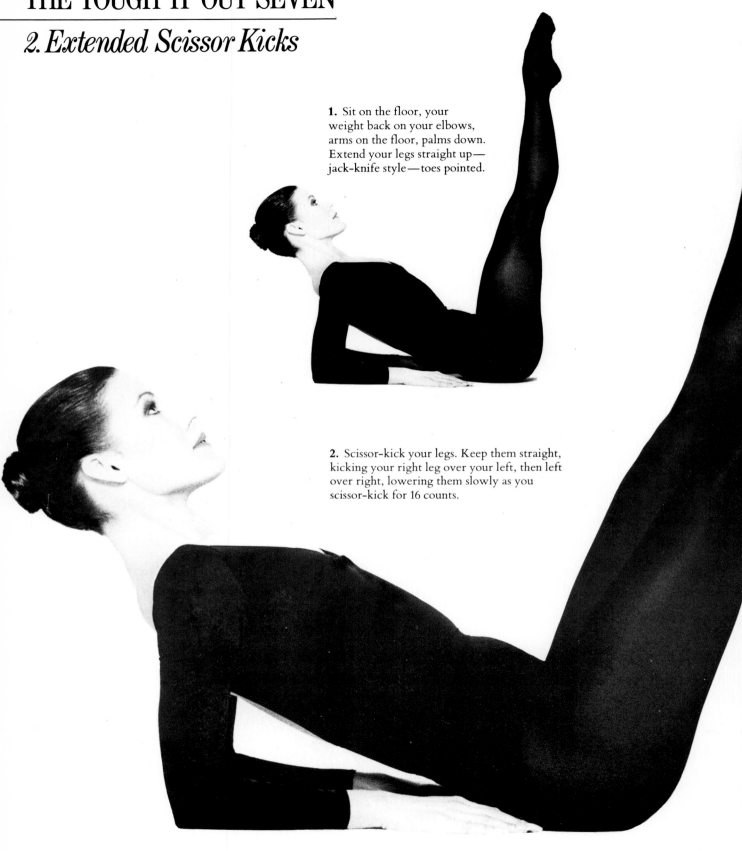

1. Sit on the floor, your weight back on your elbows, arms on the floor, palms down. Extend your legs straight up—jack-knife style—toes pointed.

2. Scissor-kick your legs. Keep them straight, kicking your right leg over your left, then left over right, lowering them slowly as you scissor-kick for 16 counts.

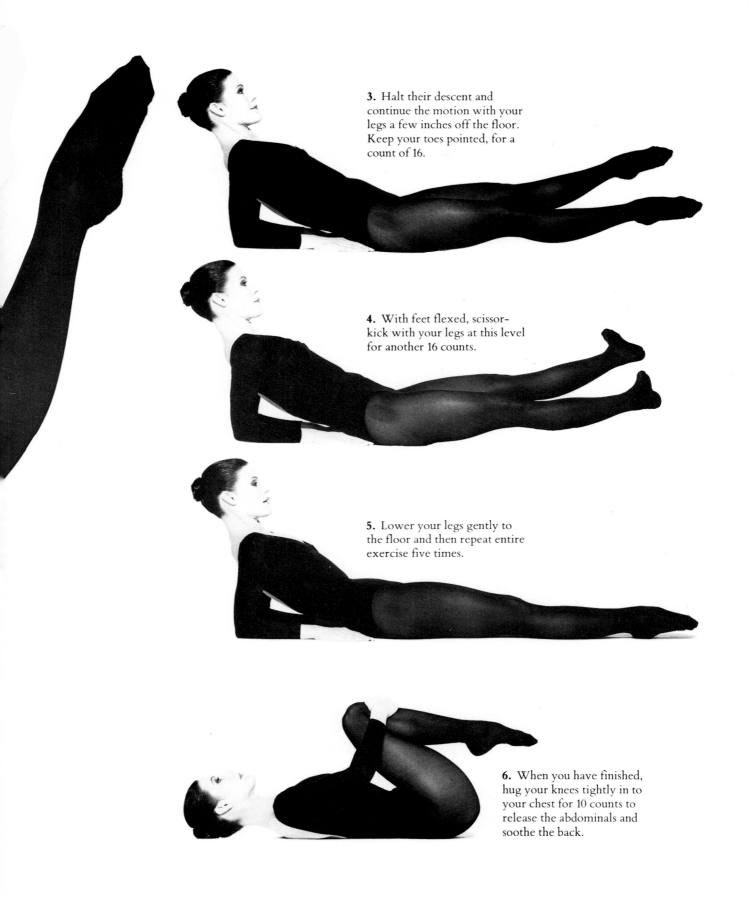

3. Halt their descent and continue the motion with your legs a few inches off the floor. Keep your toes pointed, for a count of 16.

4. With feet flexed, scissor-kick with your legs at this level for another 16 counts.

5. Lower your legs gently to the floor and then repeat entire exercise five times.

6. When you have finished, hug your knees tightly in to your chest for 10 counts to release the abdominals and soothe the back.

THE TOUGH-IT-OUT SEVEN

THE TOUGH-IT-OUT SEVEN

5. Leg Swings

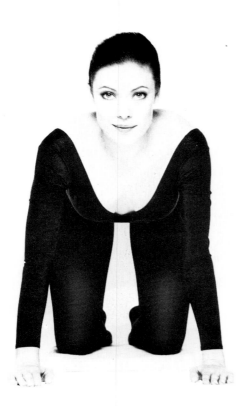

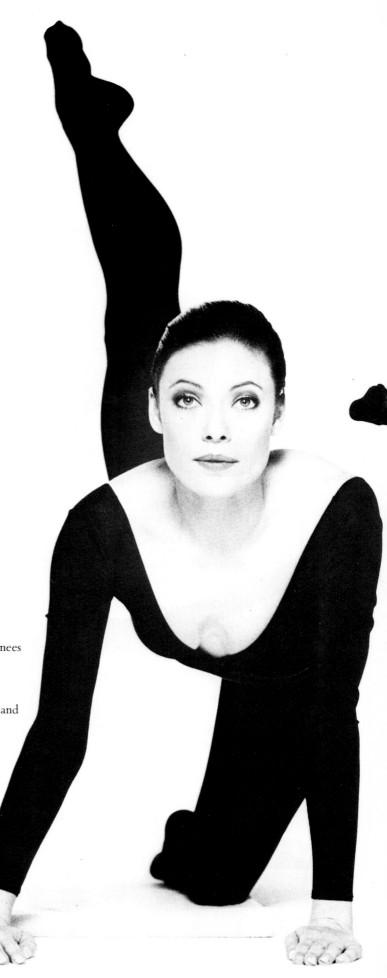

1. Kneel on all fours, your hands shoulder-width apart, knees about one foot apart.

2. Straighten your right leg behind you with toe pointed and raise it above your head, or as far as you can.

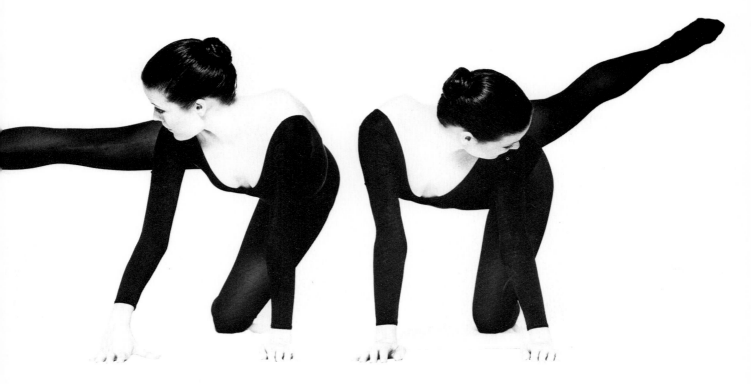

3. Swing your right leg out to the side as far as you can. Flex your foot and twist at the waist to look over your right shoulder.

4. Now stretch your foot and swing your right leg across to the left as far as you can. Twist at the waist to look over your left shoulder. Repeat 32 times with each leg.

6. Inner Thigh Lifts

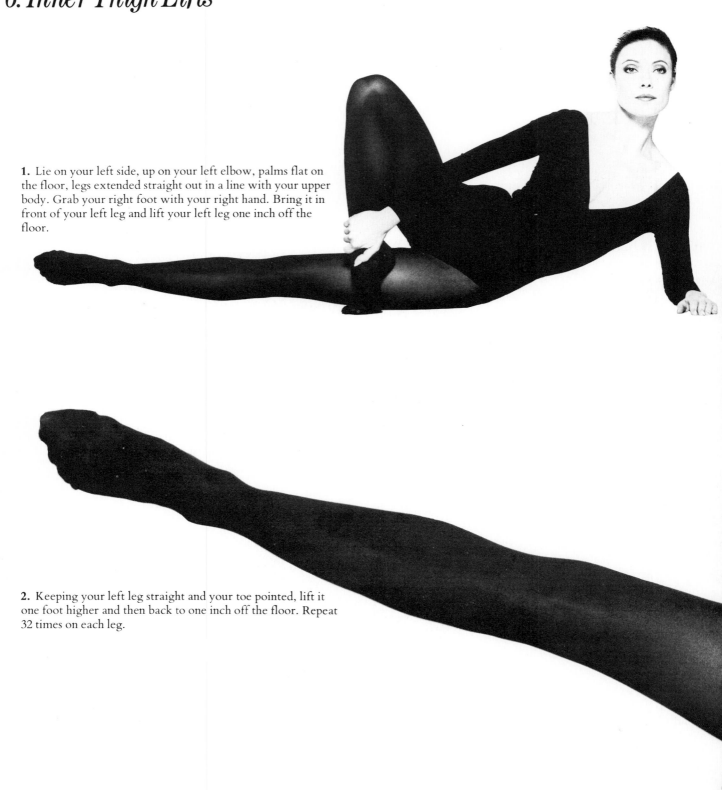

1. Lie on your left side, up on your left elbow, palms flat on the floor, legs extended straight out in a line with your upper body. Grab your right foot with your right hand. Bring it in front of your left leg and lift your left leg one inch off the floor.

2. Keeping your left leg straight and your toe pointed, lift it one foot higher and then back to one inch off the floor. Repeat 32 times on each leg.

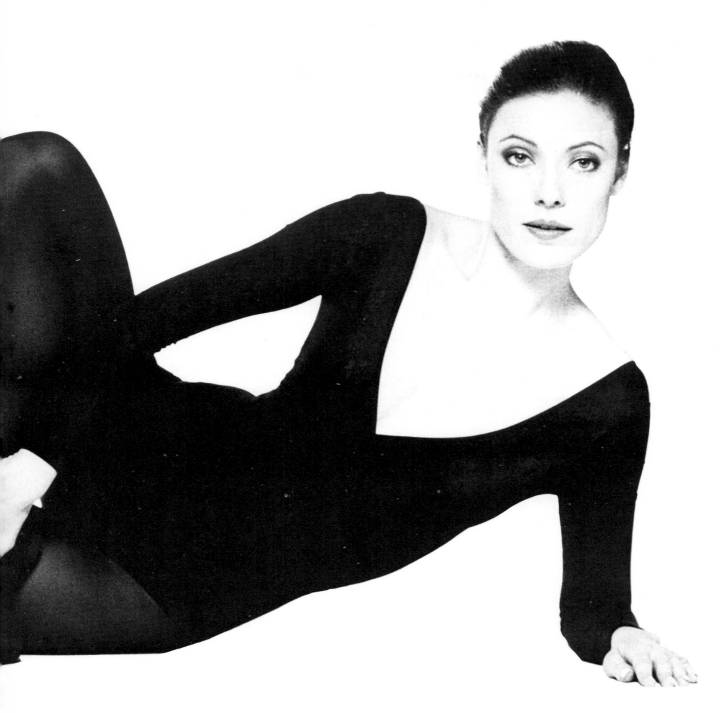

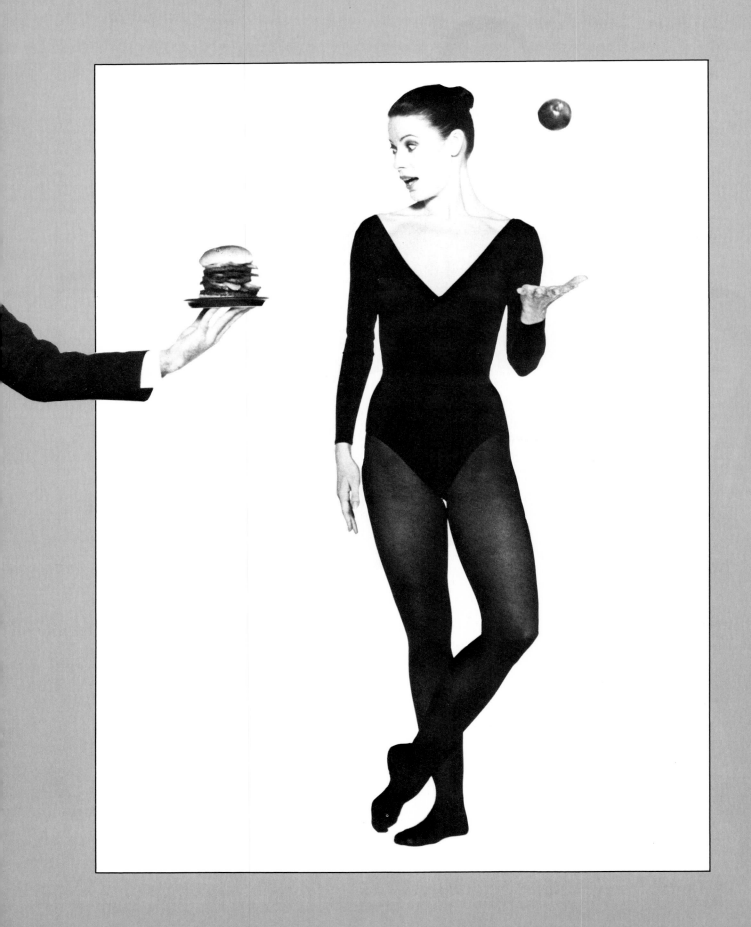

3

Nutrition & Weight Control

Nutrition & Weight Control

No book on fitness and beauty would be complete without a chapter on nutrition. But while my brother, Dr. Kevin Kain, was happy to lend a hand in writing about fitness, the subject he knows best, we thought it would make sense to go directly to a nutrition expert for information on this important subject. So impressed were we with the work of Dr. Elizabeth Bright-See, that I decided to invite her to write most of the chapter herself.

Dr. Bright-See is a nutrition consultant with H.B.B. & Associates in Toronto. She has written the recently published *Everywoman's Book of Nutrition* (with Jane Hope) and has a syndicated newspaper column on nutrition. I would like to thank her for the following chapter, which adds so much to the whole fitness picture.

What is Nutrition?

Nutrition is not magic. Good nutrition will not guarantee good health, but you can't be healthy or fit without good nutrition. Neither will good nutrition guarantee beauty, but what you eat does affect the tone of your skin, the sheen of your hair, the strength of your nails and sparkle of your eyes. It's also important for your vitality which is more likely to make you attractive than the costliest cosmetics or fashions.

We in North America are lucky. We have abundant supply of foods to provide all the nutrients we need, if we choose wisely. Being well nourished, like being fit, doesn't just happen. You have to give it some attention, particularly if you need to keep your total intake under control to watch your weight.

In this chapter we'll talk about how to get the right amount of energy, how to use it efficiently and all the nutrients that are needed for hair, skin, muscles and the rest of you.

Why do we need food?

First we need food for energy. Energy is measured in calories or kilojoules and we need it simply to keep our bodies going. While most people spend their time trying to avoid the energy in foods, you have to accept the fact that energy is basic to our survival.

How much energy each of us needs depends on how efficiently our bodies use food and on how active we are. Small differences in these two factors can make quite a difference in the amount of energy needed.

To plan your eating to get just the right amount of energy for you, it helps to know the sources of energy in our food.

Most of our energy comes from the three macronutrients, carbohydrate, protein and fat. Both carbohydrate and protein have four calories or 17 kilojoules per gram. Carbohydrates are contained in fruits, vegetables and cereal products as well as the sugars and sugary foods. Proteins are found mainly in eggs, fish, poultry, milk and meats. Some vegetables (beans and peas, especially soybeans) also contain protein.

Protein from any source may be burned for energy. We need only enough protein to replace and maintain our own body protein or 40 to 45 grams a day for an adult woman. It's not difficult to get that much protein when you consider that one egg or one-half cup of lentils has six grams, one glass of 2% or skim milk has nine grams, one-half cup of low-fat cheddar cheese has 16 grams and a three-ounce serving of most meats, fish or poultry has from 20 to 30 grams. In fact, most North Americans get nearly twice as much protein as they really need.

The average North American gets 40 percent of his or her calories from fats. Fat is the most concentrated form of energy; it has 9 calories or 38 kilojoules per gram, more than twice as much as a gram of carbohydrate or protein. Fats may not be so easy to spot in our foods. Butter, margarine and oils are obvious sources of fat. Most of the fats in our diet, however, come from hidden sources, such as ice cream, cheeses, red meats, fried foods, or mixed dishes prepared with fat.

We should cut back the amount of fat we eat to 30 to 35 percent of our total energy. Studies show that in countries where people eat a lot of fat, there is an increased rate of heart disease and cancer of the breast or colon. That doesn't mean that the fat causes these diseases; many research projects are underway to determine their exact cause. But, until the results are in, it would be wise to limit your fat intake. At the very least it is a good way to control your total calorie intake.

In some parts of the world, as much as 80 percent of peoples' calories come from carbohydrates. In North America, it's 45 percent. It would be better for our general health if as much as 50 to 60 percent of our energy came from carbohydrates, though people find this difficult to accept.

There is a fourth energy-giving substance that a lot of people forget, or would like to forget: alcohol. A gram of alcohol has seven calories or 29 kilojoules. That means that 12 ounces of regular beer has about 150 calories, a four-ounce glass of regular wine, or one and one-half ounces of gin, vodka, scotch, rye or rum has about 100 calories, so the calories can add up fast if you're not watching. You can cut down somewhat on calories by choosing light beer or light wine now on the market.

Why do people continue to eat high-fat, high-protein foods when carbohydrates are better for you? It could be because carbohydrates, particularly starches, have gotten a bad name. No one is sure how or when this started, but the first low-carbohydrate reducing diet was published in the late 1800s in England. Perhaps it was based on an observation that people who eat a lot of food also appear to eat a lot of starch. Actually, in England at that time, the upper class overate meat and fat rather than starch, and it was these people who had weight problems.

What *is* fattening is simply getting too much food or energy relative to the amount of energy you burn up; any food can be fattening if you eat too much of it. But a carbohydrate food will contribute less to our total energy intake than an equal amount of fat food.

Another misconception is that proteins are slimming. Many of the low carbohydrate diets promote protein as having some magical ability to just make the fat "melt away." That, of course, is not true. Protein has the same energy value as carbohydrates. And protein foods such as meats and milk products usually have more calories per gram because they often contain fat as well as protein.

The myth about carbohydrates may have arisen because of the effect they have on water retention. If you follow a balanced low-calorie diet, you don't lose much weight for a while. That's because as body fat is removed, your body tries to maintain it's weight by storing water. Eventually this water and its weight is lost.

On a low-carbohydrate diet water is not retained, so "magically" you start to lose weight right away. But as this is mostly water, not fat, it will all come back when you start to eat normally again.

Another diet myth is that it's possible to lose weight without reducing calories: calories don't count. Sorry, but they do, no matter where, when, how or in what foods you consume them. One pound of fat is made up of 3,500 calories that you've consumed unnecessarily.

All excess calories are stored as plain fat although some promoters would like us to believe that most women, even thin ones, are afflicted by patches of cellulite or "bad fat"—a combination of fat, water and toxic wastes—which is harder to shed than other fat. Don't believe it! Sponges, cactus fiber washcloths, horsehair mitts, cellulite "dissolving" creams, vitamin-mineral supplements with herbs, quick-result exercise programs, bath oils, massage, rubberized pants, brushes, rollers and toning lotions are among the "sure-fire" remedies that have been promoted to destroy cellulite. Special salons offer "hormone" or "enzyme" therapy, warm wax treatments and electrical muscle stimulators.

Thousands of dollars are spent each year to treat this condition, which according to the American Medical Association, simply doesn't exist. A position paper from the Medical Society of the County of New York concludes that "the truth is that fat is fat, wherever it may be located in the body."

If all fat is the same, why do some fatty areas of the body, particularly on women, look so lumpy?

Many of the fat cells under the skin can store large amounts of fat. Fibers connect the skin to deeper tissue and separate the fat cells into compartments. When we gain weight, the fat cells do not increase in number but they enlarge. The compartments of fat bulge. This produces a waffled appearance similar to the pattern of irregularities on the surface of an orange. The pattern can be seen more easily if you compress your skin lightly between your fingers.

Women have more of these fatty bulges than men because they tend to put on weight on their breasts, hips, buttocks and thighs. Men are more likely to gain weight on their stomach or abdomen; the fatty compartments beneath their skin are usually smaller than those of women and therefore do not "bulge" as much as they gain weight. In addition, women's skin is thinner and becomes even thinner and less elastic with age so the bulges are more likely to show.

How much food is enough?

We all need energy from our foods, but we don't need too much. Getting just the right balance is sometimes difficult in a society where food is always available and where it is so easy not to exercise.

Controlling our weight demands that we take a hard look at our eating habits. Those of us with a propensity to be overweight know that the yo-yo effect (20 pounds off, 15 more back on) plagues us whenever we finish the current fad diet and go back to old days.

Karen Kain, though she burns off a great deal more calories daily than the average woman, nevertheless watches what she eats: "Though I don't lose weight easily I do keep my calorie intake down," she says, "by consuming less red meat and eating fish and chicken—without the fatty skin, of course. I also enjoy steamed vegetables with grated skim cheese and herbs. I eat a lot of salads. In fact, I judge a restaurant by the quality of their salads and whether their vegetables are crunchy. Sometimes, ordering crudites—raw vegetables with a dip—is a good meal on its own."

Indeed, while North American society has long projected the ideal woman as slim, by slavishly following that ideal, we could sacrifice nutrients and ignore what our body tells us is right. The right weight is the weight at which we look and feel best.

Here is a table showing healthy normal weights for adult women.

Women of ages 25 to 59*			
Height (with 1 inch heels)	Frame		
	Small	Medium	Large
Feet Inches	lbs.	lbs.	lbs.
4 10	102-111	109-121	118-131
4 11	103-113	111-123	120-134
5 0	104-115	113-126	122-137
5 1	106-118	115-129	125-140
5 2	108-121	118-132	128-143
5 3	111-124	121-135	131-147
5 4	114-127	124-138	134-151
5 5	117-130	127-141	137-155
5 6	120-133	130-144	140-159
5 7	123-136	133-147	143-163
5 8	126-139	136-150	146-167
5 9	129-142	139-153	149-170
5 10	132-145	142-156	152-173
5 11	135-148	145-159	155-176
6 0	138-151	148-162	158-179

Reprinted with permission from Metropolitan Life Insurance Company, New York.

Karen says that her ideal weight is 115 pounds: "People are stunned I weigh that much. But dancers really go by whatever weight we feel best at. We tend to go by what we look like in the mirror rather than the scales. Everyone is so different. I'm 5 feet 7 inches tall. My body would like to be 120, but I feel best dancing at 115. If you lose a lot of weight as a dancer, it looks good on stage because lights do add pounds. But you feel awful—weak, with no energy."

You'll notice that the weight table allows us a lot of latitude: if you're 5 feet 4 inches tall, your weight range should probably be 115 to 150 pounds. This means, if you're comfortable with your body, exercise and eat properly, your ideal weight may be 135 pounds and striving to maintain 115 will only frustrate you, leaving you weak as well as unhappy! Your doctor will help you determine the best weight for you; he or she should be consulted before you undertake any diet.

Is one diet as good as another?

Hundreds of weight-control diets have been published in recent years and many of these have become best sellers. It's impossible to evaluate them all but some of them are outlined later in this chapter.

High-protein, low-carbohydrate diets such as the *Scarsdale Diet*, are very popular because you get fast, if temporary, weight loss. The other popular feature of such diets is that most people don't get hungry although the diet is low in calories. That is because substances called ketones are produced when fat is partly oxidized, or burned up. When these ketones build up in the blood, they decrease appetite. They are not believed to be harmful (except perhaps to pregnant women, insulin-dependent diabetics and alcoholics) but may give breath and urine a strange odor.

There are other diets that emphasize carbohydrates over proteins. The *F-Plan Diet* and the *Pritikin Diet* are ones that can be recommended with only a few reservations. The *Pritikin Diet* attempts to mimic the high-carbohydrate diets eaten in many parts of the world. The diet advocates increased use of whole grains, fresh vegetables and fruits, and decreased amounts of animal protein and fat, alcohol, sugar and salt. The plan also includes a healthy dose of daily exercise, but no alcohol, coffee, tea or soft-drinks.

The direction of the diet is sound, although following it to the letter means you have to prepare nearly all of your own foods. And there is no evidence that such a diet will guarantee the long and healthy life promised in the book.

The *F-Plan Diet* recommends a high-fiber intake as part of a low-calorie meal plan. The fiber helps keep you from getting so hungry. North Americans usually consume 20 grams or less of fiber a day and may find it takes a little while to adjust to the higher amount. The only problem associated with the *F-Plan* is that fiber decreases absorption of minerals, including iron and calcium. Because these are already low in the diets of many women, special attention should be given to getting at least the recommended intakes of iron (14 mg a day) and calcium (700 mg a day) if you follow this diet.

The following is a summary of the most popular diets.

Some Popular Weight-Control Diets

High-protein, low-carbohydrate diets
The majority of diets on the market, including all sorts of quick weight-loss diets, diet revolutions, and the *Scarsdale Diet*. May be high in fat. Very low carbohydrate intakes may lead to fainting spells.

The F-Plan Diet
A balanced low calorie diet that is made easier by inclusion of 30-40 grams of dietary fiber. May decrease absorption of minerals such as calcium and iron.

The Pritikin Diet
10% fat, 70-80% carbohydrate; sound idea but difficult to follow in the extreme form.

The Beverly Hills Diet
Based on a very limited selection of foods, uses mainly fruits. Unsound both in theory and in the diet prescribed.

Grapefruit diets
Also called *Mayo Clinic Diet* though no association with this famous clinic exists. The claim that grapefruit dissolves fat is not true. Some versions contain more than the recommended amount of eggs.

Liquid or powdered protein diets
Includes the *Last Chance Diet* and *Cambridge Diet*. Based on a fast, which allows small amounts of high quality protein foods and which should be attempted only in hospital. Some side effects include: dizziness, nausea, dehydration, constipation, muscle cramps, dry skin and temporary hair loss. Several deaths have been reported due to unsupervised use of this type of diet.

No single diet is ideal for everyone. Dietetic associations suggest that you ask these questions about any diet you're considering:

- Is the diet flexible? Make certain your diet allows you enough choices so that, if you need to stick to it for more than a few weeks, you can. Make certain, too, that it's the kind of diet you can follow easily if you have to eat in restaurants often. If you prefer five small meals to three large ones, choose a diet that allows you this choice.

- Is it too low in calories? A diet lower than 1000 calories daily is not advisable. Start with a 1200-calorie daily diet. A weight loss of one or two pounds per week is desirable and healthy.

- Is it nutritious and well-balanced? This is where most fad diets lose out. Some, like the banana diet, are just plain silly while others may be downright dangerous! You can get the nutrients you need and still lose weight by following Canada's Food Guide. If the diet has 1200 calories or less, use a good multivitamin-mineral preparation each day.

- Can you afford it? Steak may be less fattening than fatty hamburger but there are plenty of other nutritious foods that may better suit your budget.

- Does the diet fit in with your family's eating patterns? No sense trying to follow a diet that varies a great deal from what the rest of your family eats. If you're the meal-maker, the problem of cooking two meals (one for you, another for them) is just too much!

- Does it reflect the foods you like to eat? Some dieters become demoralized without an occasional treat—a glass of wine, a sweet or forbidden meat. Allowing occasional indulgences is more realistic than banning all forbidden foods. Your diet should consist of foods you like to eat rather than concentrating on foods you dislike or rarely eat.

Hunger is a physiological response indicating that the body needs food. But appetite, the real culprit in overeating, is a learned response to food. Some people eat more when they're upset, irritated or angry while others eat less during stressful times. Some of us have learned to clear our plates even when presented with food that's not our favorite; in the same situation our slim friends eat a little and leave the rest.

Consider the following questions. They may help you to understand the errors in eating patterns:

- Are you eating only when hungry or are there other emotions that trigger your appetite, such as anger, boredom, frustration, nervousness? Is food a reward to you? Do you eat to make yourself feel better about disappointments in your life?

- Do you snack or overeat in response to certain stimuli? For example, while watching TV, cooking for a dinner party, when the phone rings, while making the kids' lunches?

- Is your eating behavior different on certain days or at certain times during each day? Do you eat mostly from dinner on? Do you eat more on weekends?

- Where do you do most of your eating? In the kitchen while making food for others? In the TV area? At the table?

- Do you overeat alone or when you're with other people? Why? Is it boredom or social anxiety?

- Do you plan daily what you'll eat or just grab whatever is in the fridge that appeals to you at the moment?

Once you've recognized the habits that lead to overeating, next comes the battle to change them. And some are easier to change than others. If your downfall comes from snacking in front of the TV, for example, it may be quite simple to keep your hands busy with things other than food: knitting, sewing, beading, brushing the dog or painting your nails can all be done without losing track of most TV plots!

Here are a few other tips:

- The smaller the serving, the fewer the calories. Cut down on portion size—a guaranteed calorie counting method.

- Plan your meals. This may be less exciting than spontaneously cooking up a storm in the kitchen but it may be the key to helping control your weight. If you both plan your meals and shop for the required food on a full stomach, you've better chance of avoiding high-calorie foods.

- Don't skip breakfast. A good, balanced breakfast with some type of protein (milk, eggs, cheese or peanut butter) will help suppress your appetite. You will not be as likely to overeat the rest of the day.

- Cut back on high-calorie snack foods. If you live alone, don't have them in the house. If other family members consider these treats, keep them in a cupboard out of sight and away from your reach. Always store carrot sticks, broccoli florets and other raw vegetables in the fridge.

- Eat slowly. Chew your food well. Take little bites. Try putting your fork down between bites. Sip your beverage. These trite tricks really work! And don't be afraid to move the food around on your plate a lot when out to dinner.

- Substitute five knee bends for five potato chips. That old joke about pushing yourself away from the dinner table for exercise is really good advice. When you're about to reach for that cookie, run on the spot for 60 seconds. Instead of touching that leftover turkey, touch your toes 20 times. And rather than run off that chocolate cake you had for a snack, run away from the cake and save yourself the calories.

- When eating out, ask for appetizer portions for your entree, salads without dressing, foods that are steamed rather than fried and a cup of cappuccino (espresso dressed up with frothy milk topped with cinnamon) instead of dessert.

- Fill up your spice cabinet. Substitute nutmeg for butter on spinach, sprinkle curry powder on chicken, try cinnamon on a baked apple instead of cream.

  And finally, follow Karen Kain's tip:
- "I drink water throughout the day. Six glasses of water at intervals throughout the day will make you feel full, help relieve constipation and, if you choose water during coffee-break, will help cut down your daily caffeine intake."

Do I need to exercise to lose weight?

Exercise improves the function of your heart, circulatory system and muscles and may help you lose weight or prevent weight gain.

Like diets, exercise is not magic. In one hour, a 130-pound person uses 265 calories in normal cycling, 320 in walking, 520 in swimming (slow crawl), 400 to 500 in playing tennis and 850 in running. It takes several hours of strenuous exercise to burn up a pound of fat (3500 calories).

A little exercise spread over a long time may keep your joints moving and your heart pounding, but to lose fat you must achieve a certain threshold level of exercise. The American College of Sports Medicine suggests that each exercise period should use up 300 calories; anything less than this just uses up the carbohydrate stored in your muscle as glycogen and does not burn up fat. They also recommend at least three sessions a week. Fewer sessions, even if they are longer, produce little or no change in the amount of body fat.

There are several other reasons to include exercise in a weight control program. While exercise alone may not cause you to lose weight, in combination with a proper low-calorie diet, it can influence the type of weight you lose. That is, exercise decreases or eliminates the loss of lean tissue, ensuring that the weight you shed is mainly fat.

Exercise may help you stick to your diet. It can serve as what behavioral scientists call an "incompatible behavior," that is, anything during which you can't eat. It's difficult to munch during a tennis game or a swim. In addition, if you exercise strenuously enough, the lactic acid that builds up in your blood actually suppresses appetite.

What other nutrients does my body need?

Energy and planning how to get just the right amount of energy is very important. But for all-round good health, we need many nutrients. Some of these are necessary for the proper use of our food as energy, others are essential for bones, hair, skin and eyes.

The energy materials—carbohydrates, protein, fat and alcohol—are just like gas or oil for our furnace. We don't get any benefit from them unless they are metabolized or "burned" in our bodies.

Converting these fuels to energy is a rather complicated process requiring many micronutrients, that is, vitamins and minerals. If you do not have the pep and energy you would like, it could be because one or more of these critical nutrients are missing and the energy in what you eat is not fully released.

Two of these key nutrients, iron and folic acid (also called folacin or folate), are essential in transporting oxygen to all your cells where the fuels will be "burned" or oxidized. They are also ones likely to be lacking in the diets of North American women.

Iron is the essential factor in hemoglobin. Without iron, oxygen cannot attach to the hemoglobin and, therefore, it can't be transported to all the body's tissues.

Menstruating women need about 14 milligrams of iron a day. This is sometimes hard to get because there are only a few really good food sources of iron, such as liver and red meats. Beans baked with molasses, chicken, turkey and enriched or whole grain breads and cereals are fair sources. Iron from animal products is generally better absorbed than that from plant products.

If you just can't eat one serving of these high iron foods once a week and several servings of other sources every day, you should consider using a supplement—ferrous sulfate, gluconate or fumurate. Ten milligrams a day should be sufficient unless your doctor diagnoses severe iron-deficiency anemia. Don't waste your money on "organic" or "natural" iron.

Folic acid is also necessary for hemoglobin synthesis. (So are protein and vitamin B_6, but you're likely getting enough of these unless you're following an imbalanced vegetarian diet.)

It's easy to know the sources of folic acid when you remember that the name comes from the word foliage. Therefore, most green leafy vegetables, especially spinach, brussel sprouts, cabbage, broccoli, asparagus and green beans are good sources along with cantaloupe, kidney, liver, soybeans, wheat bran and wheat germ. You need 200 micrograms of folic acid a day and unless you avoid all these types of foods you're probably getting all the folic acid you require. That may not be true if you are pregnant or using oral contraceptives, "the pill." In both cases, absorption of folic acid is decreased, so supplements of up to 400 micrograms a day are often prescribed.

Other key nutrients in energy utilization are the B-vitamins—thiamin (B_1), niacin (B_2), riboflavin and pyrodoxine (B_6). Deficiencies of these are rare in North America and are usually found only in people with very low food intakes or following an unusual or restricted diet. These vitamins are often promoted as a means of giving the user super energy or for helping to overcome stress. That is not the case. Very small amounts of these vitamins are enough and any extra will simply be excreted in your urine.

In fact, if you take enough riboflavin (which is yellow) you can see it turn the urine yellow.

The most abundant nutrients of the body are protein, found in muscles, organs and the framework of bones, and calcium found mainly in the bones. These two substances together help make up our basic body structure. Protein has already been mentioned as a source of energy, but the really major role of protein is in building and maintaining our muscles, organs and bones.

The majority of North Americans eat more than enough protein every day. And they get high quality protein, that is, the type that is used most efficiently in building body protein.

Recently, many people are trying to reduce the traditional sources of high quality protein in their diets, that is, meat, milk and eggs. Vegetarian and semi-vegetarian diets, which are becoming more popular, may introduce some nutritional problems that were hitherto seen only in the poorest parts of Africa and Asia. Rickets, vitamin B_{12} deficiency and kwashiorkor, diseases common to developing countries, cause quite a stir when they show up in North America.

New vegetarians are people who have recently adopted a meatless way of eating. They often belong to religious and philosophical groups that are based on Eastern thought. What they don't have is the long experience and tradition that makes vegetarianism a reasonable and nutritionally sound alternative in other parts of the world.

A vegetarian diet may be nutritionally adequate if it is well planned. But it takes a bit of know-how to do that planning. There are several types of vegetarianism and each has its special problems. People who merely avoid red meat (i.e., semi- or partial-vegetarians) can easily eat as well as non-vegetarians if they substitute poultry, fish or other protein food for meat.

Lacto-ovo-vegetarians eat a non-flesh diet. They don't use meat, poultry, fish, or seafood, but eggs and milk products can be used. This type of diet can be nutritionally adequate for any healthy adult or child.

Lacto-vegetarians use milk, but not eggs. The elimination of eggs is a significant change. Eggs, like meat, supply good quantities of iron in a form that is easily absorbed. The iron in beans, peas, whole grain, or enriched cereals, prunes and molasses, which they substitute for eggs, is not so readily absorbed. Eating these plant foods together with a food high in vitamin C, however, will help increase the amount of iron absorbed.

Total vegetarians or vegans avoid all animal food. Some may further restrict their diet to mainly fruit or raw food. The fewer types of food in a diet, the more difficult it is to include all of the required nutrients.

The most severe vegetarian diet is the Zen Macrobiotic. All we want to say about that one is don't try it. It has proven to be lethal for several people.

In our society we associate meat, milk, and eggs with protein. We often forget that that essential nutrient is also found in plant foods, especially beans, peas, cereals and nuts. Both the amount and quality of protein in plant foods are lower than in animal foods. The exception is soy protein. Soy products, such as tofu and soy milk, are an excellent source of protein in vegetarian and non-vegetarian diets alike.

The quality of vegetable proteins can be increased by using them in combinations with each other or with eggs or milk, if these are used. For strictly plant combinations, the basic rule is to eat a grain with a legume—for example, rice and beans. The combination of the two foods gives a higher quality protein than found in either alone.

Plant foods are generally rich in vitamins and minerals. However, there are four nutrients that may not be present in adequate amounts in a strict vegetarian diet. These are vitamin B_{12}, vitamin D, calcium and iron.

There are no practical plant sources of vitamins B_{12} and D. Vitamin B_{12} can be obtained in small quantities in milk or eggs, or in the form of a supplement, as B_{12} fortified soymilk or soy protein "meat" products. Seaweed or fermented soy are sometimes used as a source of vitamin B_{12}, although right now no one knows how much vitamin B_{12} they contain. You should not rely on them. A better source of B_{12} is nutritional or food yeast. This contains more B_{12} than other yeasts (Brewer's, baker's, or live) because it is grown on a solution that is rich in this vitamin.

Vitamin D can be produced in the skin when it is exposed to sunlight. The amounts supplied this way may be enough for an adult, but not for a growing child. Some soy milks are fortified with vitamin D and these should be used for growing children.

The major source of calcium in the North American diet is milk. The best replacement in a strict vegetarian diet is fortified soy milk, which supplies both calcium and vitamin D. Regular, large servings of dark green vegetables (except chard, spinach, and beet greens in which the calcium is tightly bound to a substance called oxalic acid), legumes, almonds or sesame seeds may supply enough calcium for adults.

Adults may benefit from a partial or total vegetarian diet. Vegetarians tend to be leaner than non-vegetarians. They also usually have lower serum cholesterol levels. They may be less likely to develop osteoporosis (bone demineralization) but this is still debatable. The diet is usually low in fat and cholesterol, and high in fiber and does not contain a lot of high calorie-low nutrient foods.

Bones, like muscles, are constantly being broken down and rebuilt. If we're supplying our body with sufficient calcium all the calcium in our bones is replaced every five years. If not, the result is osteoporosis, the condition of severe bone demineralization.

Until we reach adulthood more calcium enters the bones than leaves them. But at middle age the loss of bone mineral speeds up and out-distances the growth of new bone. If this continues over a long time, we have smaller, more fragile bones. Persistent back pain, "shrinking," and the familiar dowager's hump are all signs of this condition.

Women of all ages should be concerned about osteoporosis. Bone demineralization is a slow process starting in middle age. It usually cannot be detected in the early stages; 30 percent of the bone must be lost before it can be seen by an X-ray examination. After menopause, calcium is lost from the bone more rapidly because of decreased estrogen production.

While the exact causes of osteoporosis have not yet been found, some studies have shown that osteoporosis can be halted or sometimes reversed by diets containing 1500 mg of calcium a day or about twice the recommended intake of calcium. The average calcium intake of women in the United States is 450 micrograms a day.

The build-up or removal of calcium from bone is influenced by a number of other factors: hormones, diet and exercise. Estrogen is sometimes used in the treatment of osteoporosis but the results have not been completely successful. Fluoride and vitamin D therapy are also being tried.

Protein may also be important. We do need the protein to form the framework for the bones. On the other hand, too much protein seems to inhibit the depositions of calcium in the bones.

Bones, like muscles, become stronger when they are used or stressed. Regular exercise promotes strong bone development. Extreme inactivity—for example, during confinement to bed—leads to severe bone demineralization.

There is a limit to every good thing of course, and some dancers and athletes develop their muscles so much that they are too strong for their bones. The result is fine breaks in the bone called stress fractures. Most people will never reach this extreme, but we all have a vested interest in maintaining our bones by diet and exercise.

While osteoporosis may be developing slowly without our knowing it, there is one evidence of calcium problems that is more obvious: leg cramps. Many people, even if they don't exercise strenuously, suffer from leg cramps. This happens to women particularly during pregnancy. The level of blood calcium affects muscle function so an imbalance of calcium in the diet, that is too little calcium in relation to phosphates (which come primarily from meats), sometimes causes leg cramps. You may find that a good calcium supplement (calcium lactate, fumerate or gluconate) is useful in relieving this problem.

What nutrients do I need for beautiful hair, skin, nails and eyes?

Our skin, hair, nails and eyes were developed from nutrients we got from foods and these same nutrients are needed continually to keep everything healthy and attractive. Deficiencies of particular nutrients may show up on these external tissues, but we should remember that problem skin or hair can be the result of a variety of causes other than a poor diet. If you have such problems, do try to improve your diet. If that doesn't work, consult a qualified medical specialist.

Many nutrients are essential for healthy skin. A deficiency of vitamin A causes hard rough skin; too little vitamin C leads to red spots, particularly on the arms and legs. Diets low in protein or many of the B vitamins cause rough, peeling skin. Fortunately deficiencies severe enough to cause these problems are rarely seen in North America. And contrary to what you may have read, extra amounts of these nutrients will not help skin that has been damaged by wind, water, sun or harsh cosmetics.

One skin problem often blamed on diet is acne. But all studies show that food has little, if any, role in this condition. However, if it seems that one particular food causes acne to flare up, avoid it. Most of the foods that people say increase their acne—fried foods, soft drinks and chocolate—can be eliminated from the diet without the loss of important nutrients.

Dull, dry, thin hair that is losing its color and is easily pulled out may be the result of severe protein deficiency, but excessive bleaching will cause some of these same problems. Severe calorie restriction is one of several reasons that all of a person's hair may fall out, a condition called alopecia.

Hair analysis is being erroneously promoted as a means of diagnosing a variety of nutritional problems. The only nutrients that may be checked in the hair are minerals, but the amount of minerals there are may depend on how the hair was prepared, what type of shampoo, hair color or permanent you had, the fineness or coarseness of your hair, your gender. As yet, there are no standards of how much of each of the minerals should be in the hair or how they relate to the amounts of minerals in the rest of the body. In short, hair analysis will tell you nothing significant about your health.

It's said you can see a person's soul through his eyes. That may or may not be true, but you can certainly tell from a person's eyes whether they've had enough sleep or too much to drink. Eyes can also sometimes reveal if their owner is badly nourished.

Dry, dull eyes with redness and white spots are a sign of vitamin A deficiency. Of course, the first sign of a deficiency of this nutrient is night blindness, that is, difficulty in seeing in dim light. A lack of riboflavin or pyridoxine can result in redness and cracks at the corners of the eyelids. White rings or small yellowish lumps around the eyes are symptoms of hyperlipidemia (high blood cholesterol and triglycerides). This serious condition is fairly common in North America and should receive prompt medical attention.

The mouth can also tell a lot even when not used for talking. White or pink breaks at the corner of the mouth, red or swollen lips, and a purplish tongue indicate a riboflavin deficiency. A scarlet, raw and swollen tongue may also result from a deficiency of riboflavin.

Spongy, bleeding and receding gums mean a deficiency of vitamin C. And, of course, everyone knows that tooth decay is caused by using too much sugar at times you can't clean your teeth.

Changes in nails can indicate a deficiency of iron. They become spoon-shaped, brittle and ridged. Nails may stop growing with a severe protein deficiency (hair will, too) but taking gelatin will *not* make your nails stronger. Gelatin is a poor quality protein. It does contain a type of amino acid present in nails, hydroxyproline, but that particular amino acid has to be made in the body. Any of it in the diet will be used for energy rather than protein synthesis.

Are there other important nutrients I should include in my diet?

So far we've discussed the high-profile nutrients, those for which we can easily see a role. There are, however, several other essential nutrients that have important, if less obvious, roles. Some of their more important functions are listed later in this chapter.

One item on the list, fiber, is not truly a nutrient, but it is a food substance that is important for our health. Many different materials, mainly cellulose, hemicellulose, lignin and pectin, make up fiber. What they have in common is the fact that we have no enzymes to digest them. They pass on to the large intestine where some of them are digested by the colon bacteria and others are eliminated.

Although most people think only of wheat bran when they hear the word fiber, fibers are found in all plant foods, fruits, vegetables and unrefined cereals and breads. Wheat fibers are well known for their laxative effects; oat fibers (which contain a lot of gums) may prove to be useful for decreasing serum cholesterol and for controlling blood glucose in people with diabetes.

On the average, North Americans get 20 grams or less of fiber a day. Many studies show that they should probably get 30 to 40 grams from a variety of foods.

Protein
In addition to the functions already discussed, it helps regulate the water and acid-base balance of the body and is also part of enzymes, hormones and antibodies needed to fight infections.

Vitamin A (Both vetinol and carotene)
Essential for healthy organs, such as bladder, lungs and stomach as well as healthy skin.

Thiamin (Vitamin B₁), Riboflavin (Vitamin B₂)
They help maintain a healthy nervous system.

Niacin (Vitamin B₃)
Necessary for normal growth and a healthy nervous and gastrointestinal system.

Pantothenic Acid
Helps heal wounds; necessary for using energy.

Pyridoxine (Vitamin B$_6$)
Needed for protein synthesis for bones, muscles, etc.

Vitamin B$_{12}$ (Colbalamin)
Along with folic acid, is necessary for healthy red blood cells. Also helps maintain the covering that protects nerves.

Folic Acid or Folacin
Also needed for formation of white blood cells.

Vitamin C (Ascorbic Acid)
Essential to the production and maintenance of collagen, the protein-base structure of bones, skin, teeth, etc.

Vitamin D
Needed for the normal absorption of calcium.

Vitamin E (Tocopheral)
Is an antioxidant, but its exact role is not yet clear.

Calcium
Mainly found in bones and teeth but it is also necessary for maintaining muscle tone.

Iron
As already discussed, it is the essential component in hemoglobin.

Zinc
Needed for a normal sense of taste. May aid wound healing.

Fiber
Bulking agent that promotes normal bowel function.

The Whole Picture

Probably few of you start off your day by saying: "Today I'll eat 50 grams of protein and 800 mg of calcium." Tables of recommended intakes of the nutrients we've discussed are available but are not very practical in our day-to-day eating.

That is why the recommended nutrient values have been translated into foods, the stuff we all know about. This translation is called *Canada's Food Guide,* or in the United States, *The Basic Four.* They remain the best and simplest sets of rules for maintaining healthful eating habits.

The Guide is simply a logical grouping of foods according to the nutrients they contain. Breads and cereals supply protein, fiber, minerals, and B vitamins. The Guide recommends that we use three to five servings of whole grain or enriched bread products each day. Fruits and vegetables are excellent sources of vitamin C and vitamin A. They also contain fiber and some minerals and B vitamins. The Guide recommends at least two servings of vegetables in a total intake of four or five servings of fruits and vegetables each day.

Canada's Food Guide*		
Food Group	**Servings**	**Examples of one serving**
Milk and milk products *Children up to 11 years* .... 2-3 *Adolescents* .... 3-4 *Pregnant and nursing women* .... 3-4 *Adults* .... 2 *Skim, 2%, whole, buttermilk, reconstituted dry or evaporated milk may be used as a beverage or as the main ingredient in other foods. Cheese may also be chosen.*		240 ml (1 cup) milk, yoghurt or cottage cheese 45 g (1½ ounces) cheddar or process cheese *In addition, a supplement of vitamin D is recommended when milk is consumed which does not contain added vitamin D.*
Meat and alternatives	2	60 to 90 g (2-3 ounces) cooked lean meat, poultry, liver or fish 60 ml (4 tablespoons) peanut butter 250 ml (1 cup) cooked dried peas, beans or lentils 80 to 250 ml (⅓-1 cup) nuts or seeds 60 g (2 ounces) cheddar, process or cottage cheese 2 eggs
Bread and cereals *Whole grain or enriched. Whole grain products are recommended.*	3-5	1 slice bread 125 to 250 ml (½-1 cup) cooked or ready-to-eat cereal 1 roll or muffin 125 to 200 ml (½-¾ cup) cooked rice, macaroni, spaghetti
Fruits and vegetables *Include at least two vegetables. Choose a variety of both vegetables and fruits—cooked, raw or their juices. Include yellow or green or green leafy vegetables.*	4-5	125 ml (½ cup) vegetables or fruits 125 ml (½ cup) juice 1 medium potato, carrot, tomato, peach, apple, orange or banana

*Adapted from Canada's Food Guide, *Health and Welfare Canada, 1982.*

Milk and milk products, of course, are our main supply of calcium. They also give us protein, riboflavin, vitamin A and, in fortified products, vitamin D. Children up to eleven years need two to three servings. Teenagers and pregnant and lactating women need three to four servings. Other adults need only two.

The so-called meat group also contains eggs, fish, beans and peas, and other sources of good quality protein, minerals, and vitamins. Two servings a day is adequate for most people.

Canada's Food Guide also recommends that within each group we select a variety of foods every day. Studies have shown that a monotonous diet is more likely to be deficient in nutrients.

The recommended daily nutrient intakes and *Canada's Food Guide* are designed to help us avoid deficiencies of protein, vitamins and minerals. Clinical signs of such deficiencies are very rare in this country and will remain so as long as we follow the Guide.

The Guide was not designed to recommend energy intakes, but diets based on it (and not supplemented with cakes, candy or alcohol, or other high caloric foods) supply between 1000 and 1400 calories per day. If you need more than that, use more servings from each group or add other foods.

The last word on nutrition should go to Karen: "Even dancers with no previous weight problem have to learn good nutritional habits. We travel a lot, eat at irregular hours and dine out at restaurants or snack in our hotel rooms. If you're not aware of proper nutrition, it's easy to make the wrong food choices. Some dancers are so worried about their weight that they eat very little—another nutritional hazard.

"But when you rely on your body—and of course, all of us do—you need to fuel it properly. And once you know a little about nutrition and become more aware of which foods contain what, you can make sound nutritional choices. You also learn that some of your favorite foods are really good for you, too."

Recipes

Even though I don't have as much time as I would like to spend at home and in the kitchen (and let's face it, how many of us do these days!), I do love to cook whenever I can. Over the years I have found hundreds of recipes that meet all my requirements: the dishes are low in calories but filling, nutritious, and above all, delicious and fun to make and serve.

Here is a selection of twenty of my favorite recipes. Since most people already have the perfect recipe for roast beef and steak (foods that I don't eat terribly often anyway), I didn't include those here. I'd like to introduce you to a lighter way of eating. And an easier way of cooking—all of these dishes can be prepared simply.

Cold Zucchini and Watercress Soup

A touch of curry powder makes this an intriguing soup—as does the combination of green vegetables.

6 leaves Boston lettuce
6 small to medium size zucchini
3 leeks, sliced thinly
1 bunch watercress
2 tbsp. (30 ml) curry powder
4 cups (1 L) chicken broth
1 cup (250 ml) milk
½ cup (125 ml) plain yogurt

Rinse, dry and trim the vegetables. Chop coarsely. In large pot, bring chicken broth to boil. Turn down heat to medium and add leeks to cook 10 minutes. Add zucchini, lettuce and watercress and cook 10 minutes. Add 1 tbsp. (15 ml) curry powder. Stir. Cool to room temperature. Puree mixture in blender or food processor. Add milk. Stir. Chill thoroughly. Serve in bowls topped with yogurt sprinkled with the rest of the curry powder. Serves six to eight.

Gazpacho

Low-cal, nourishing and refreshing, serve this summer or winter—each bowl garnished with a dollup of plain yogurt.

1 20 oz. (625 ml) can stewed tomatoes
1 cucumber, seeded
1 stalk celery, coarsely chopped
1 green pepper, coarsely chopped
1 cup (250 ml) tomato juice
3 cloves garlic, crushed
2 tbsp. (30 ml) soy sauce
1 small onion, chopped
2 tbsp. (30 ml) olive oil
1 tbsp. (15 ml) red wine vinegar

In a food processor or blender, puree stewed tomatoes and put in large bowl or pitcher. Add tomato juice. Blend chopped vegetables and add to tomato mixture. Add garlic, soy sauce, oil and vinegar. Season with fresh pepper. Serves six to eight.

Seafood Broth

This light broth is pretty to look at, nourishing and perfect for a lunch (just add a salad) or for a soup course in a larger meal. Use only fresh seafood, but to keep costs down slice scallops thin and chop shrimps.

5 cups (1.25 L) of fish stock (or chicken broth)
1 cup (250 ml) dry white wine
2 carrots, sliced julienne (very thin strips)
2 stalks celery, sliced julienne
1 small onion, sliced julienne
½ lb. (225 g) scallops, sliced very thin
½ lb. (225 g) large shrimps, peeled and deveined
½ tsp. (2 ml) tarragon
½ tsp. (2 ml) chervil
½ tsp. (2 ml) basil

In a large pot bring to a boil the fish stock and wine. Add the vegetables and seafood, turn down heat to medium and poach for 3 to 5 minutes or until seafood is just tender. Transfer vegetables and seafood to soup bowls. Add herbs to broth. Stir. Pour over vegetables and seafood. Serves four to six.

The Best Chicken Salad Ever

This is not only a great solution to leftover white chicken meat. It's also incredibly tasty and an unusual luncheon dish.

2 chicken breasts, skinned, deboned, cooked and cut into
bite-sized pieces
1 cup (250 ml) plain yogurt
½ cup (125 ml) pine nuts, toasted in oven
½ cup (125 ml) watercress, chopped
½ cup (125 ml) dried apricots, cut into small pieces
½ cup (125 ml) lemon juice
salt and pepper to taste

Put apricots in lemon juice and set aside for 30 minutes or until fruit has absorbed all juice. In a bowl, combine chicken, apricots, pine nuts, and watercress. Toss with yogurt to coat evenly. Salt and pepper to taste. Chill. Serves two.

Pasta Primavera

By now, this once unusual dish has become commonplace—but it's no less delicious than when first introduced as a fresh departure from traditional spaghetti with meat sauce. While it has to be made at the last minute, you can blanche the vegetables well ahead of time—then reheat to serve.

1 bunch broccoli, sliced
2 small zucchini, sliced
6 green asparagus spears, sliced
1 cup (250 ml) green peas, frozen
1 cauliflower, broken into flowerets
1 cup (250 ml) mushrooms, sliced thinly
2 tbsp. (30 ml) unsalted butter
¼ cup (60 ml) chopped parsley
2 cloves garlic, crushed
1 cup (250 ml) tomatoes, chopped
2 tbsp. (30 ml) basil
¼ cup (60 ml) pine nuts, toasted in oven
1 lb. (450 g) spaghetti or linguine
1 cup (250 ml) chicken broth
⅓ cup (80 ml) cream
⅔ cup (160 ml) grated Parmesan cheese

In large soup pot, bring about six quarts (5.7 L) of water to a boil. Drop in vegetables, except for mushrooms and tomatoes. Cook for 1 minute only. Remove to drain with slotted spoon. In frypan, melt butter. Sauté garlic. Add tomatoes and mushrooms and cook 3 to 5 minutes. In pot where vegetables cooked, drop pasta into boiling water and cook according to directions. Drain. Toss vegetables with tomato mushroom mixture. Mix into pasta. Keep warm. In frypan, bring chicken broth to boil. Reduce by one-third. Stir in cream, parsley and basil. Toss sauce throughout pasta and vegetable mixture. Toss in pine nuts and Parmesan cheese. Serves six to eight.

Vegetarian Moussaka

This traditional Greek dish made with eggplant and lamb gets a delicious meatless twist thanks to Toronto vegetarian cooking school teacher Nettie Cronish. Serve with green salad, crusty bread and full-bodied red wine.

3 medium eggplants
2 lbs. (900 g) mushrooms, sliced
3 tbsp. (45 ml) unsalted butter
1 large onion, chopped
2 cloves garlic, crushed
6 oz. (190 ml) tomato paste
¼ cup (60 ml) chopped parsley
1 tsp. (5 ml) basil
1 tsp. (5 ml) tamari (an aged soy sauce found at Japanese
*   supermarkets or health food stores)*
dash of pepper
½ tsp. (2 ml) cinnamon
¼ cup (60 ml) dry red wine
½ cup (125 ml) fresh wheat germ
½ cup (125 ml) grated cheddar or Parmesan cheese
4 beaten eggs or 12 oz. (375 ml) pureed tofu
½ cup (125 ml) unsalted butter
½ cup (125 ml) whole wheat flour
2 cups (500 ml) warm milk
¼ cup (60 ml) Parmesan cheese, grated

Preheat oven to 350°F (177°C). Bake sliced eggplant on lightly oiled cookie sheet 15 minutes. Melt 3 tbsp. (45 ml) butter in large skillet. Sauté onion and garlic until transparent. Add mushrooms and sauté for 2 minutes. Add tomato paste, parsley, basil, tamari, pepper, cinnamon, red wine. Simmer until liquid is absorbed. Add wheat germ, cheese, eggs or tofu. Mix well. Remove from heat. In another saucepan, melt ½ cup (125 ml) butter over low heat. Whisk in flour—mixing constantly to make a roux. Slowly whisk in warm milk. Whisk constantly until thickened. Butter a large casserole. Make layers of eggplant slices followed by mushroom mixture. After two layers of each, top with white sauce. Sprinkle with ¼ cup (60 ml) Parmesan cheese. Bake 30 minutes covered; 15 minutes uncovered. Serves six to eight.

Baked Sea Bass

1 large 3 to 4 lb. (1.4 to 1.8 kg) sea bass, scaled and
*   cleaned but head left on*
½ cup (125 ml) all-purpose flour
1 tsp. (4 ml) freshly ground pepper
4 tbsp. (60 ml) unsalted butter
1 clove crushed garlic
1 cup (250 ml) clam juice or fish stock
3 tbsp. (45 ml) minced parsley
3 tbsp. (45 ml) chopped basil
3 tbsp. (45 ml) chopped rosemary

Preheat oven to 375°F (190°C). Pepper the fish and coat with flour. Melt butter in large skillet. Add garlic. Sauté fish over medium-high heat for 3 or 4 minutes on each side—until the fish skin begins to brown. Reserve skillet. Carefully transfer fish and pan juices to large baking dish. Bake fish uncovered for about 35 minutes—or until flaky at the bone. In the skillet where the fish was fried, bring clam juice or fish stock to a boil, scraping up any bits from the bottom of the pan. Add herbs. Reduce to ¾ cups (190 ml). Fillet fish into portions and pour sauce over each. Serves four to six.

Ceviche

This Mexican-inspired dish is perfect for those who hate to cook since it cooks, over days, in its own juices. Make a batch weekly, then eat it for light meals or add it to salads.

1½ lb. (680 g) fresh bay scallops, thinly sliced
1 cup (250 ml) lime juice
½ lemon, squeezed
peel of ½ lemon, thinly sliced
1 red onion, thinly sliced
½ cup (125 ml) sliced green pepper
1 tbsp. (15 ml) dried chili peppers
½ tsp. (2 ml) dried oregano
2 tbsp. (30 ml) chopped fresh coriander leaves (optional)

Layer all ingredients, except juices, in bowl. Pour over lemon and lime juice. Cover. Refrigerate 12 to 24 hours. Serve with twist of lime on lettuce leaves. Serves six to eight.

Poached Salmon

The great thing about poached salmon is that you can make it ahead to serve cold—with a selection of garnishes and, if you like, a simple sauce made from yogurt, chopped dill, parsley and cucumber. If you don't have a fish poacher, use a large skillet.

12 cups (2.8 L) water
1 lemon, sliced
1 large onion, sliced
3 sprigs parsley
6 sprigs dillweed
3 cloves garlic, crushed
1 bay leaf
6 fresh salmon fillets or one large tail section or centre cut
    weighing about 4 lbs. (1.8 kg).

Bring water, lemon, onion and herbs to boil in fish poacher or skillet. Reduce to simmer. Gently poach the salmon in broth until it is done. (The flesh will become firm and its color lighten.) Remove from broth. When cool, refrigerate until ready to eat. When ready to serve, granish with fresh watercress, lemon wedges, quartered hard-cooked eggs and the following sauce. Serves six.

Yogurt-Dill Sauce

1 cup (250 ml) plain yogurt
½ cup (125 ml) chopped dillweed
1 cup (250 ml) chopped English cucumber
½ cup (125 ml) chopped parsley

Mix all ingredients well. Service with fish.

Tabouli with Prunes

This combination of grain and fruits is delicious. Full of fibre, it can be served any time. Make it the night before to let the flavors blend.

1 cup (250 ml) bulgar (cracked wheat)
1½ cups (375 ml) boiling water
1 cup (250 ml) dried pitted prunes, chopped
1 tsp. (5 ml) salt
1 cup (250 ml) parsley, chopped
½ cup (125 ml) green onions, chopped
½ cup (125 ml) tomatoes, seeded and chopped
4 tbsp. (60 ml) fresh lemon juice
2 tbsp. (30 ml) fresh mint, chopped
1 tsp. (5 ml) fresh basil, chopped
pepper to taste
lettuce leaves

Combine bulgar, boiling water and salt. Let stand until water is absorbed by wheat. Add the rest of the ingredients except the lettuce leaves. Cover and chill. Serve over lettuce leaves. Serves six.

Red Cabbage Salad

A tasty nutritious way to put fibre in your diet. Serve this during a summer barbecue or in winter with a sandwich supper.

½ head red cabbage
1 tsp. (5 ml) salt
1 small onion, peeled and chopped
½ cup (125 ml) red wine vinegar
2 apples, peeled, cored and chopped
½ tsp. (2 ml) caraway seeds, crushed

Shred cabbage. Place in bowl. Sprinkle with salt and let stand 30 minutes. Drain. Put in bowl with apple. Combine rest of ingredients and pour vinegar mixture over cabbage and apples. Refrigerate 3 hours. Serves four.

Real Bran Muffins

1 stick corn oil margarine, softened
¾ cup (190 ml) dark brown sugar
½ cup (125 ml) dark thick molasses
5 eggs
2 cups (500 ml) milk
3 cups (750 ml) coarse wheat bran
2 cups (500 ml) all-purpose flour
1 tbsp. (15 ml) baking powder
1 tsp. (5 ml) baking soda
1 tsp. (5 ml) salt
1½ cups (375 ml) Sultana raisins
½ tsp. (2 ml) cinnamon
½ tsp. (2 ml) nutmeg
½ cup (175 ml) walnuts, chopped

Preheat oven to 425°F (218°C). Put margarine in bowl with sugar, molasses, eggs and milk. Mix thoroughly. Add bran and half the flour. Mix again. Add baking powder, baking soda and salt to the rest of the flour. Slowly, add this flour mixture to the bowl, mixing all the while. Add raisins, spices. Mix well again. Divide mixture into muffin tins. Bake 20 minutes or until knife inserted comes out clean. Immediately top with walnuts. Let cool. Makes about two dozen.

Brunch on the Run

Breakfast really is the most important meal, so if you're in a hurry or not too interested in food this early try this nutritious alternative. It's also good enough to have for lunch: just add a healthy side salad.

1 cup (250 ml) orange juice
1 cup (250 ml) pineapple juice
½ cup (125 ml) plain yogurt
1 ripe banana, broken up
4 ripe strawberries
1 tbsp. (15 ml) brewer's yeast
1 tbsp. (15 ml) toasted wheat germ
4 ice cubes

Combine all ingredients in blender and blend until fairly smooth. Serves two.

Cheesy Apple Bread

Wholesome, nutritious, delicious. What more can I say?

½ cup (125 ml) shortening
½ cup (125 ml) sugar
2 eggs, beaten
1½ cups (375 ml) fresh Spartan apples, peeled and grated
1½ cups (375 ml) sharp cheddar cheese, grated
1¾ cups (440 ml) flour
⅓ cup (80 ml) wheat germ
1½ tsp. (7 ml) baking powder
½ tsp. (2 ml) baking soda
½ tsp. (2 ml) salt
½ tsp. (2 ml) cinnamon
¼ tsp. (1 ml) nutmeg

Preheat oven to 350°F (177°C). Add sugar and eggs. Beat until light and fluffy. Blend in apples and cheese. Sift dry ingredients together. Add to apple mixture. Mix lightly. Turn into well-greased 8" x 4" x 3" (20 cm x 10 cm x 7.5 cm) loaf pan. Bake for 50 to 60 minutes. Serve warm. Makes one loaf.

High Protein Punch

Here's a drink that's perfect for breakfast, lunch or the four o'clock slump.

1¼ cup (310 ml) ice water
1 tbsp. (15 ml) powdered milk
1 tsp. (5 ml) protein powder
2 tbsp. (30 ml) unsalted cashews or peanuts
2 tsp. (10 ml) sunflower seeds
1 tsp. (5 ml) honey
dash cinnamon
dash nutmeg
1 orange twist

Put first two ingredients in blender and blend 5 seconds. Slowly add the next ingredient, blending about 3 seconds between each addition, until you've added everything but the spices. Sprinkle with cinnamon and nutmeg. Pour into tall glass. Add orange twist. Serves one.

Tomato Cooler

Try this, with a muffin, for a nutritious summer snack or light lunch.

1 cup (250 ml) tomato juice
2 tbsp. (30 ml) lemon juice
1 tsp. (5 ml) Worcestershire sauce
½ tsp. (2 ml) soy sauce
fresh pepper

Combine all ingredients and serve over ice. Add celery tree to garnish and a dollup of fresh plain yogurt as a float.

Low-Cal Viennese Iced Coffee

1 tbsp. (15 ml) instant coffee
1 tbsp. (15 ml) powdered cocoa
2 cups (500 ml) cold skim milk
1 tsp. (5 ml) vanilla
6 ice cubes

Combine coffee, cocoa, milk, vanilla and ice in blender. Blend until fairly smooth. Pour into two glasses.

Oranges in Red Wine

This is a sophisticated yet easy to make dessert. It's perfect as a summer cooler or as a light ending to a winter casserole. Serve chilled, and for special occasions, with freshly whipped cream.

1 cup (250 ml) water
1 cup (250 ml) dry red wine
1 inch (2.5 cm) long piece of cinnamon stick
1 inch (2.5 cm) long piece of vanilla bean
1 lemon, thinly sliced
6 large navel oranges, peeled and sliced
1 tbsp. (15 ml) orange rind, cut into slivers

In a saucepan, combine water, wine, cinnamon, vanilla and lemon. Bring to a boil. Turn to low and cook 15 minutes. Put oranges and orange rind into bowl. Pour wine mixture over. Let cool to room temperature. Refrigerate 4 to 6 hours. Serves four to six.

Karen Kain Chantilly

This dessert was named in my honor by the Food Advisory Division of Agriculture Canada. Not only is it delicious, but it only contains about 135 calories per serving!

Meringues:
8 egg whites
¼ tsp. (1 ml) cream of tartar
2 cups (500 ml) sugar
1 tsp. (5 ml) vanilla

Beat egg whites with cream of tartar until soft peaks form. Gradually beat in sugar, beating after each addition until soft peaks again form. Add vanilla and beat until stiff peaks form. Then, line a baking sheet with greased foil. Using a piping bag or two spoons, shape meringue rings about 3 inches (7 cm) in diameter and 1⅛ inch (3 cm) high. Bake at 250°F (120°C) until set, 1 to 1½ hours. Turn off heat and let stand a further hour. May be stored up to a month in freezer. Do not thaw before filling. Makes about 25 meringues.

Filling:
6 cups (1.5 L) sliced fresh strawberries
¼ cup (50 ml) sugar
1 cup (250 ml) whipping cream
2 tbsps. (25 ml) icing sugar
1 tbsp. (15 ml) kirsch
OR 1 tsp. (5 ml) vanilla

Combine strawberries and ¼ cup (50 ml) sugar. Whip cream, gradually adding icing sugar and kirsch, until stiff. Fill each meringue with ¼ cup (50 ml) strawberry mixture and 2 tbsps. (25 ml) whipped cream. Garnish each serving with a strawberry slice. May be held for up to half an hour at cool room temperature. Makes 25 servings.

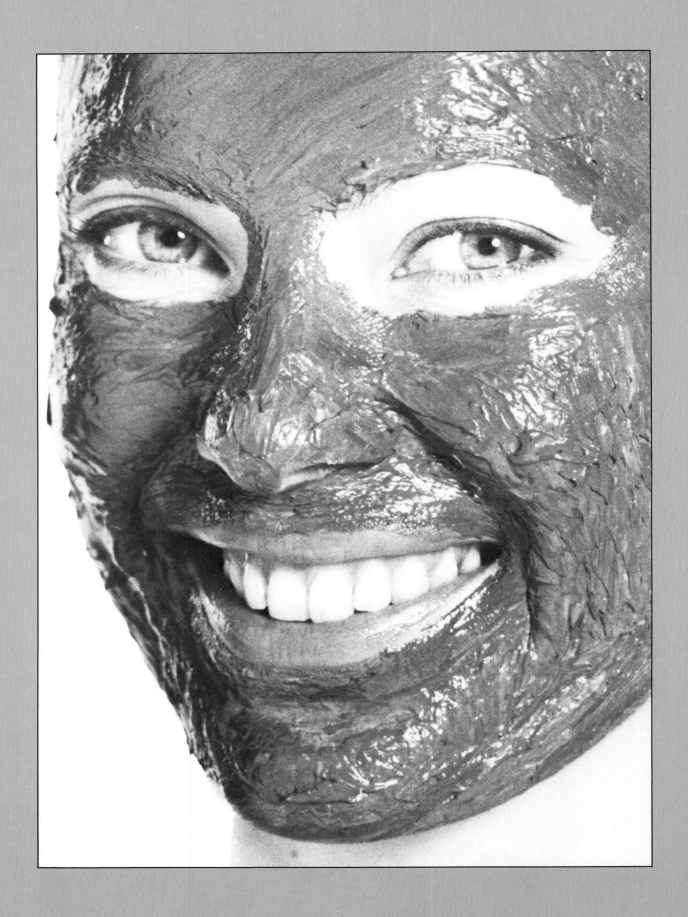

5
Skin

Skin

What is the body's largest and most amazing organ? The answer to this question, of course, is the skin. Few people think of it as an organ, but it is. And few people realize how incredibly efficient the skin is in its many functions. What other organ, for example, does all the following?

- Covers and protects the whole body. As with other animals, our skin protects our bodies by functioning as a barrier against outside elements.

- Produces essential Vitamin D. When our bodies are exposed to daylight or sunlight, an inactive precursor of Vitamin D present in the skin is converted into the vitamin and absorbed into the blood.

- Controls body temperature. Nothing cools your body better than a swim, or warms you up faster than extra clothing next to your skin. Temperature changes are really achieved through the skin's messages to its capillaries. Is incredibly elastic. The skin's elasticity is something pregnant women know only too well. But we can also appreciate the skin's elasticity in its ability to accommodate our body movements. When we bend our knee, for example, the skin stretches, then contracts back into shape.

- Replenishes itself daily. Our skin sloughs off old top cells twice daily: in the morning and early in the afternoon. These are good times to cleanse and reapply makeup.

Because it works so hard, protects so much and presents our "package" to the outside world, skin is well worth looking after. Like the rest of the body, it demands respect, daily attention and sometimes special care.

The Sun

Most experts would agree that the sun is one of the skin's worst enemies. Chronic exposure to sunlight over many years may lead to premature aging—meaning that the skin looks older because through constant exposure it loses its elasticity and becomes dry and wrinkled. As well, there's a direct relationship between skin cancer and continual exposure to sun, particularly for fair-skinned people.

Now doctors are also warning sun-sensitive patients who take certain drugs (such as tetracyclines) to put off that summer-time tan because the combination of drugs with sun may induce certain allergic reactions.

And, of course, there's sunstroke, which can be serious, even fatal. But more than any of the above, what most of us suffer is the occasional sunburn. It hurts. And despite what many people think, it doesn't turn into a tan. As the burn fades a bit, a little of the tan we acquired during our burning begins to show through. To alleviate mild sunburn, apply vinegar or 3% sodium bicarbonate on a wet cool cloth held gently against the burn; follow with a calamine lotion. For serious burns accompanied by fever, chills and nausea, consult a doctor.

How can you get the most of the sun without burning? Remember these things:

- When the skin is exposed to the sun's ultraviolet rays, it produces melanin, a brown pigment that contributes to skin color and that acts somewhat as a shield against damaging rays. Know your skin. Some of us have fewer melanocytes and produce melanin more slowly and so burn more quickly.

- Learn to choose your tanning hours more wisely. Since the hours of most intense sunlight (these are the most direct and harmful rays) are between 11 A.M. and 3 P.M., it's essential to tan before or after—particularly if your skin is sun-sensitive, if you're vacationing in countries close to the equator, or if you're at the beach or on a ski slope where, because of the reflection from the water or snow, we burn more easily. Plan your tan slowly, even if you have to start it in late spring. Begin each season with no more than 15 to 25 minutes in the sun, depending on your skin type and the sun's intensity that day.

And even if your complexion is dark, use a suntan preparation. They include lubricating moisturizing agents, which minimize drying out of the skin, and sunscreen, which actually protects against burns. To find the best sunscreen protection, study each product's sunscreen index to match its protection to your skin's needs: obviously, the higher the protection factor, the more your skin will be spared harmful rays.

Moisture

Along with staying out of the noon-day sun, proper skin care also requires moisturization. In hot or cold dry weather, at home in winter, on windy days, the skin loses water through evaporation. As a result, it's thirsty.

To keep my skin fresh and radiant, I drink plenty of water daily. My fridge is always stocked with a few bottles of mineral water and some lemon, sliced. I try to choose waters with low or no sodium content. (Soda water, while it's very popular, contains salt and even makes some people thirsty.)

Doctors recommend that we drink at least six glasses of water a day—not including the water we consume in beverages such as tea or in foods such as tomatoes. Water, besides fighting skin dehydration, also aids in the elimination of wastes and helps to flush out toxic body materials. Though most of us drink water straight from the tap, in the last decade bottled mineral waters have become popular in North America. They vary in their claims—some come from springs reputed to cure everything from tuberculosis to arthritis. And because they come from different geographical locations, the mineral content of these waters also differ.

There are now a dozen or more imported and domestic bottled waters on the market (including Perrier, Evian, San Peligrino, Ramlösa, Montclair and Mont Blanc). When trying them, you'll notice subtle differences between them in taste, due to their mineral contents. Some beauty experts also recommend that you spray bottled water onto the face to boost the skin's moisture level.

As far as moisturizers go, suffice to say that you best experiment with many products before settling on one that does the job for you. Skin care is extremely controversial: some experts suggest that certain vitamins and other nutrients when added to face-care preparations actually work to rejuvenate and protect. Others, however, stress that creams containing vitamins, collagen or hormones do little or no good and that such claims have no scientific basis.

Whatever moisturizer you choose, plan to use it often. No matter what products claim, a moisturizer can't really penetrate further than the skin's outermost layer and, due to this restriction, it can't put moisture back into the skin for very long.

The chief function of moisturizers is to slow down the rate of moisture loss by offering a protective film. And remember, too, to use moisturizers on more than just your face. Hands, feet, knees and elbows need extra moisturizing because they're subject to calluses, rough red spots and chapping.

Even if you don't have to worry about removing heavy stage make-up like I often do, removing make-up of any kind is essential, not only for personal hygiene but because nothing looks worse than leftover make-up.

But here again, our judgement is challenged constantly in ads that claim one product cleanses better than another. Since each of us have different skin types and since each product tries to distinguish itself by having ingredients other products lack, experimentation, again, is the only way to determine the best product that will cleanse your skin without leaving too greasy or gritty a film. Beware of products that are exorbitant in price: while price sometimes reflects quality, often it does not. There are plenty of beautiful faces that rely on common cold creams, even soap.

Generally speaking, however, soap defeats and dries out the skin and, for the most part, contains no special ingredients to cleanse away stubborn make-up particles. Some are really too harsh for your face, so if you prefer to wash with water, try some of the lotion-type wash-off cleansers designed to be lathered up, then rinsed off. But if your make-up is heavy, or your face is rarely without it, do consider a good cleansing cream because its ingredients dissolve the waxes, pigments and oils contained in make-up.

The Facial

Here's what I do every evening before going to bed. It's a relaxing mini-facial that is also the best way I know to keep my face clean and properly moisturized. You'll need to tie back your hair, find a comfortable chair in front of a lighted mirror and have on hand: a supply of cotton balls, cleanser, toner or astringent and moisturizer.

First Step: Cleansing

1. Pour or scoop a little cleanser into the palm of one hand.

2. Using the fingers of your other hand, dot it all over your face.

3. Using your fingertips, gently work in the cleanser to cover the entire face (take special care not to irritate the eyes) down to the underchin and up to the hair-line.

4. Taking fresh cotton balls, gently remove the cleanser (and with it the make-up and grime) being especially careful around the eyes. Use light, gentle strokes. Change cotton balls frequently.

Second Step: Toning

1. Apply toner after cleansing is complete. Dampen cotton balls with toner.

2. Brush gently, smoothly over entire face except for eyes and mouth areas. (Some toners are so harsh, sensitive areas will sting.) Your face should tingle, not burn.

Third Step: Moisturizing

1. Squeeze or pour some of the moisturizer into the palm of one hand.

2. Using the fingers of the other hand, dot the moisturizer generously over the face.

3. Moisturize forehead with fingertips using strokes that start at the bridge of the nose and go upward and outward toward hairline.

4. In a circular motion, massage moisturizer around eyes and mouth.

5. Apply moisturizer to cheeks by using smooth gentle strokes upwards from the jaw to the temple.

6. Moisturize neck, too: using vigorous long strokes, spread the moisturizer with your fingertips from the base of the neck to the jawbone.

Home-Made Face Brews

Today, face masks are made with many different ingredients, each one promising a particular benefit not found in the others. As convincing as they sound, however, most experts say the only real benefits to face masks are their cleansing effect on the skin and the fact that they increase blood flow to the skin. The result makes you feel refreshed and your skin smooth to the touch.

There are many commercial face masks available—some of which you scrub off because they're made of fatty ingredients such as vegetable oils or wheat germs and others which you peel off because the applied mask, when left to set, turns into a kind of second skin because of its rubber or wax base. My favorites, however, are cleansing masks you can make in your kitchen, apply to your face, then, if you like, eat the leftovers.

Oatmeal Mask

Add enough warm water to ½ cup of raw oatmeal to form a thick paste. Spread on your face and neck and allow to dry. Leave on for 30 minutes. Rinse off with cool water.

Cucumber Pick-me-up

Peel and seed one medium cucumber. Puree in blender or food processor. Add 1 tsp. dried mint. Pat on face. Leave on for 15 to 20 minutes. Rinse off with cool water.

Yogurt Spread

Combine ½ cup plain yogurt, 1 tbsp. Brewers' yeast, ½ tsp. honey, 4 drops rosewater. Spread over face. Leave on 20 minutes. Rinse off with warm water.

Problem Skin

Even those of us who take good care of our skin are occasionally troubled by minor skin problems such as red patches or whiteheads. To help distinguish the minor skin problems from major ones requiring medical attention, consult the following:

Abscess

When a pimple or boil becomes inflamed and infected, pus forms. Abscesses on skin may be caused by bacteria or a hair follicle. When especially painful or large, visit your doctor. When small, apply hot poultices to try to bring abscess to a head. Use a sharp sterile needle to release the pus. Squeeze abscess gently. Dress with antiseptic cream.

Acne

The condition, which begins with blocked sebaceous glands, is further complicated by inflammation and infection and is fairly common during puberty. Doctors generally agree that acne sufferers should wash frequently with an anti-bacterial soap. Acne creams may also be prescribed. Consult a doctor.

Blackheads

They're not black because of dirt, but rather because they're compiled of keratin, which turns black upon exposure to oxygen. Because blackheads are caused by too many keratin and sebum cells blocking the sebaceous gland exit, there's nothing you can do to prevent it. Try steam, squeezing the blackhead, washing with warm water and leaving alone. Ignore or camouflage with make-up. If excessive, visit a skin clinic for a professional facial.

Broken Capillaries

If you have tiny capillary blood vessels showing through the surface of the skin (usually on the cheeks or thighs), you've probably inherited the tendency. Though you can't prevent it, you can cover it up with make-up (make sure you moisturize the area, too). If the broken capillaries are very noticeable, or seem to be getting worse, consult a doctor.

Chapping

Most common in the winter when hands and face are exposed to dry winds and bitter cold, chapping includes dryness, scaling and roughness and sometimes small painful cracks in the skin. To protect against it, moisturize vulnerable skin areas. To treat it, apply hand cream every half-hour, wear lip salve and keep hands out of water.

Freckles

These are small groups of the cells that produce melanin, the skin's pigmentation. When exposed to further sunlight, freckles often increase in number. You can use a sunscreen if they bother you, or you can cover them easily with make-up.

Rashes

While a rash may be nothing more than too much sun on a particular day, it could also signal an allergy. So try to recall what you ate, wore or did before the rash started and consult your doctor. Welts or hives on the skin is most certainly an allergic reaction. Get help as soon as possible. If you've a history of rashes and know what they're from, chances are your doctor will have recommended lotions, creams, even an antihistamine to calm them faster.

Red Skin Spots or Patches

High progesterone levels the week before menstruation may account for some, but other causes may include acne, eczema, psoraisis or other skin conditions. Because diagnosis demands a trained eye, consult a doctor.

Whiteheads

These tiny, white rounded and raised spots, usually on the face, are sebaceous cysts that get stuck in the glands. You can leave them alone, or, if large, prick the skin over the whitehead with a sterile needle and gently squeeze out. Cleanse skin with antiseptic when finished.

Wrinkles

When the skin's collagen disintegrates due to too much sun or because of age, wrinkles begin to appear. Short of cosmetic surgery, there's nothing to be done to prevent them. The tendency to developing wrinkles or not depends very much on heredity. If your parents have young-looking skin, chances are you will, too.

MAKE-UP
The Karen Kain Face

Even though I've learned a lot about make-up from working on the stage and in front of cameras, I decided to let an expert show you how it is best applied. Steve Marino is a Toronto make-up artist and he helped me with the following make-up session.

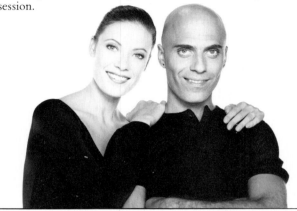

Because my skin is sensitive, delicate and a little dry, Steve applied a protective moisturizer, containing collagen, to my face. He also applied an eye cream under my eyes where the skin is especially sensitive.

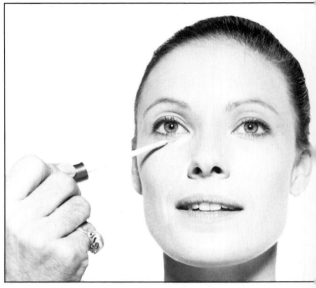

1. A light concealer (sometimes called an erase stick) is applied just around my nostrils where there's a bit of discoloration, and under my eyes where it is dark. After every application of make-up, this concealer should be blended into the skin with the fingers—beginning under the eyes and working inwards towards the nose.

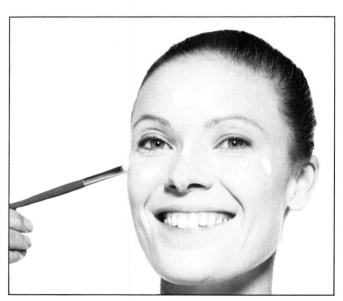

4. In highlighting, the reverse of shading, a highlight cream (two or three times lighter than the base used) is applied down the middle of my face, to the top of my cheekbones and to the bridge of my nose. This will detract somewhat from the square shape of my face and focus instead on the center of my face.

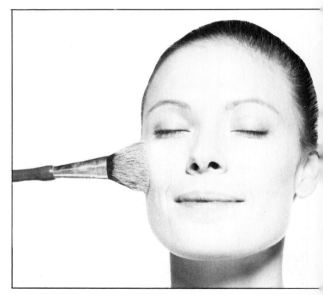

5. Powder sets the make-up and prevents a shiny face. Steve applies a translucent powder with a brush using out and downward motions (If you have oily skin, use powder in the same colors both for shading and highlighting.)

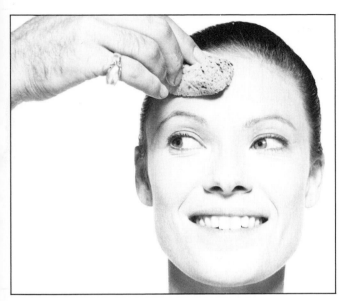

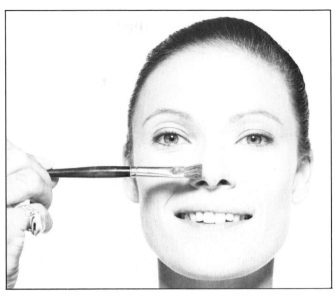

2. A liquid moisture base is applied with a damp sea sponge using down and outward motions. Because my skin is a little dry, this liquid moisture base contains a slight amount of oil.

3. In shading, a brown cream is applied with a brush to cast an extra shadow that will "restructure" certain facial features. Some people do this to change a too-square face or a double chin. Here, Steve puts some shading touches to the sides of my nose.

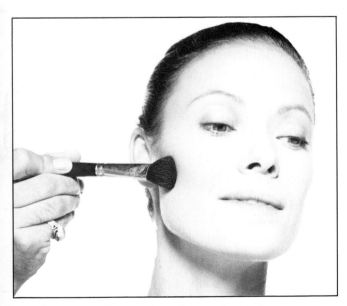

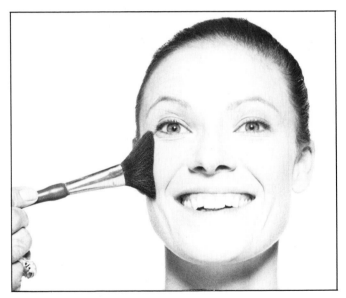

6. A "contouring" process is used to emphasize the cheekbones. To apply, find the hollow underneath the cheekbones, and, starting from near the ear brush the color (a little darker than the blush but in the same color family) under the cheekbones in a line.

7. Blush is applied by first sweeping the color where the contour on my cheekbones begins. Then the color is swept onto my cheekbone with a natural bristle baby brush to buff in and blend color lines. (Always use the same family of color for lips, eyes and cheeks. Color charts are available at most make-up counters.)

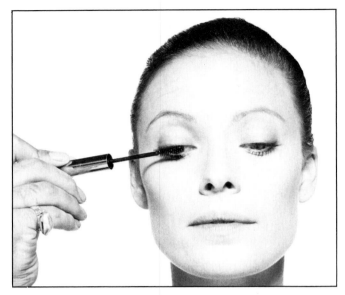

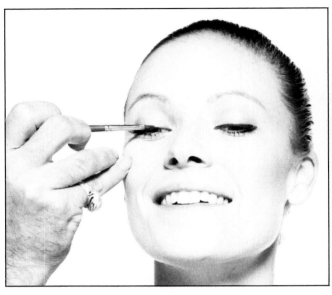

8. To give an open-eye look, my eyelashes are curled. Mascara is applied.

9. Eye-liner is applied to the top and bottom of my eye, close to the lashes but not too thick. Use a color that's close to your hair color and blend in the liner so it's not too severe.

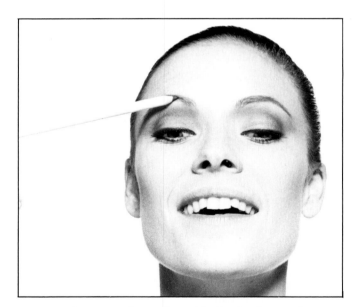

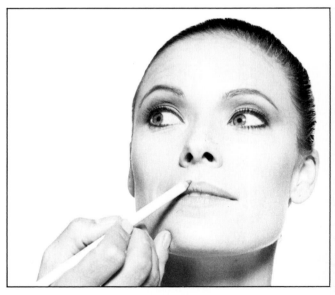

12. An eyebrow pencil is used to add a few hairline strokes because my eyebrows are sparse. If your eyebrows are thick or uneven, pluck stray hairs for a clean smooth line.

13. A lip liner is used to correct the shape of my mouth and hold my lipstick in place. We use a color in the same shade as the lipstick I will apply, and outline my mouth as closely as possible to its natural shape.

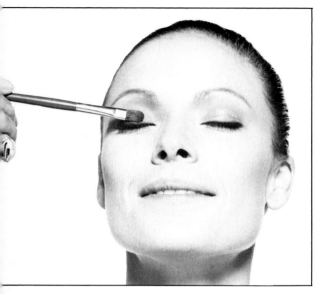

To apply shading to my eyes, my eyelid crease is contoured
th the darkest eye shadow color we're using. Next, the
or is blended back and forth along the crease to tone down
harsh line made with the sponge tip applicator. The lid
or is applied and buffed with a brush.

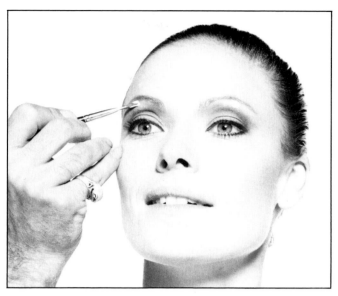

11. An off-white matte shade is used to highlight my brow
bone. Then, a brown shade is used for the crease, green for the
lid, and cream for the brow.

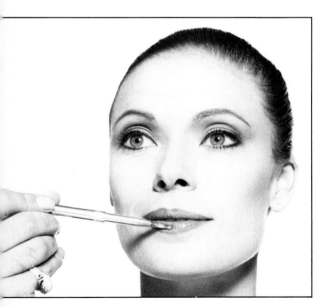

A lip brush is used to fill in the lips with lipstick. Then the
s are blotted with tissue and finished with lip gloss.

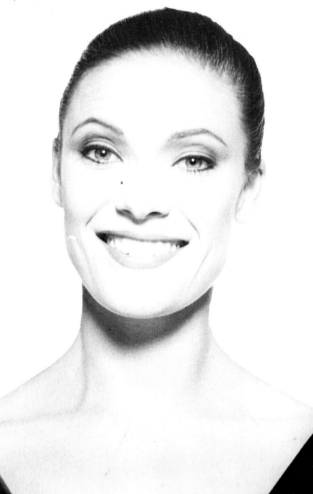

Hair

If you've ever waited for a short haircut to grow back in, you'll remember it seems like it takes forever for hair to grow. How surprising, then, to learn that the hair root is the fastest-growing organ in the whole body. Hair on the scalp grows on the average .035 millimeters a day, about ½ inch per month, and to keep up this demanding activity (our hair is really the end of a continuous process by which hair cells grow, mature and die) our bodies need to be fit to properly nourish the cells required for hair production.

When we're unfit, under stress or recuperating from an illness, our hair may grow more slowly for a time, or appear less healthy. And though we normally lose anywhere from 20 to 100 hairs per day, during times of bodily stress, such as after having a baby or an anaesthetic, or over an extended period of time of taking certain drugs, hair loss may be more than usual or noticeably thin. Because hair growth is related to hormonal actions, some women develop signs of baldness during menopause when oestrogen levels change. But oestrogen therapy, under a doctor's care, usually restores hair growth to its normal pattern.

Melanocytes, the same cells that produce skin coloring, are also responsible for hair color and are located at the tip of the hair follicle, under the scalp. But your hair color is determined by heredity—though unlike the color of your skin, which is the same forever, hair color can be altered significantly through aging (grey or white hair) or coloring.

In fact, what best distinguishes hair from other body organs is its extreme versatility. Because the hair on our heads is not living, we can cut it, curl it, color it and, in doing so, change the way we look—every month or two if we so choose. And thanks to today's highly trained stylists, safer and more sophisticated methods of coloring and curling, our hair is one of the few parts of our body whose care we can entrust to someone other than ourselves.

Even so, it's important to know what hair care products are all about—their claims and what it is they really can do. Remember, the natural condition of your hair reflects your general state of health, so whatever hair care products you choose, they have only a cosmetic effect.

Shampoos

Today, shopping for the product that in the 1950s was pure mild hair detergent has become as enticing and confusing as shopping in a supermarket. Supplements of Vitamin E, protein, balsam and a dozen other ingredients are now added to shampoos, each brand suggesting that the secret to beautiful hair is unlocked by washing with the particular blend of ingredients inside its bottle. But since no nutritive value is actually absorbed by the hair follicle, which lies under the scalp, suffice to say that most claims are superficial and do little more for hair than grandma's recipe of adding egg yolk to a favorite shampoo or mixing vinegar in the rinse water. Still, keeping your hair clean and shiny is important to hair care, so shampoos, like bars of soap, have become essential hygiene products.

While you may derive instant satisfaction from matching your dry, normal or oily hair to a shampoo made specifically for your particular hair type, many experts recommend baby shampoos, which, for most people, adequately cleanse the hair without irritating the sensitive scalp area or robbing it of moisture.

How often you shampoo depends entirely on your lifestyle and the condition of your hair and scalp. For example, you may want to wash your hair daily if it tends to be greasy or if you live in a smog-filled city or work out vigorously and often. But many experts caution against overwashing (more than twice weekly) normal hair as shampoos and hair driers can rob the hair and scalp of essential oils and moisture.

Dry hair may be helped with a mild shampoo, followed by a dry-hair conditioner and regular trimming of split ends. Grandma used to alleviate this condition by rubbing warmed olive oil into the hair and today's hairdressers offer hot oil treatments to temporarily seal the scalp and hair against further moisture loss while also coating the hair with oil. But some experts say oil treatments for dry hair are nonsense in that you need such a strong shampoo to clean your hair after the treatment that the process defeats the purpose!

Dandruff, caused by an over abundance of dead keratin cells on the scalp's outer layer, is usually stopped by using anti-dandruff shampoos. But such shampoos containing selenium, a scalp irritant, should be used not more than once every two weeks or so lest they promote rather than cure the condition. (Continual itching, scales or red patches on the scalp should be checked by your doctor.)

Conditioners

Since hairs, on the average, live two to six years, it's well worth remembering that conditioners do more to keep your hair in line than in shape since hair, unlike other body organs, is not alive. For appearance's sake, however, conditioners are worth considering for the simple reason that they make hair more manageable. For example, most cream rinses and conditioners contain ingredients that stabilize the alkalinity of tap water and, in doing so, tame flyaway static-charged hair. As well, conditioners containing oil or waxes that are not water soluble, leave a fine coating on the hair (used too often, this also leads to greasy hair) which, when applied to an average scalp's 120,000 hairs, provides body and substance and disentangles hair for easy combing.

Permanents

A perm operates by breaking down the molecular structure of the hair to rearrange its pattern from straight to curly. Its advantages, of course, are cosmetic in that naturally straight hair that's been chemically moulded into a new shape holds a hair style longer and liberates one from having to depend on unattractive and uncomfortable curlers. As well, a perm can add more volume to thin limp hair and, because it lifts hair away from the scalp, helps to combat the greasies.

The disadvantages can out-weigh the advantages for some. Perms done professionally are expensive and if done on one's own can be touch and go—too frizzy or too limp unless you're experienced. More importantly, using a perm on bleached or damaged hair can cause it further damage—even breakage. The harsh ingredients in perms can irritate sensitive scalps. And since a permanent is permanent, at least until your hair grows out, you'd better be sure you like the change in appearance it delivers.

Color

In coloring the hair, a chemical film is applied to the hair shaft and is left on long enough to remove the hair's pigment and replace it with a new tint. To do this properly requires the mixing of two solutions: an oxidant to develop the color, and an ammonia with a dye (the ammonia opens the hair shaft so that the dye can penetrate the core). Permanent dyes, because of their strength and ingredients, may cause allergic reactions in some people—hence the sensible advice to always perform a patch test on the inside of the arm a few days before applying a permanent dye to a whole head of hair.

The advantages of permanent dyes? A softer, lighter or darker shade than your own or a dramatic entirely new color. Disadvantages include possible allergic reactions, getting a color you don't like, the expense of having it done professionally (a trained colorist combines experience, judgement and technique) and the revolving hairdressing-salon door problem: once your roots begin to show, it's back for more of the same. If you firmly believe that blondes have more fun, you'll have to bleach your hair to become one. Unlike permanent dyes, which add color to the hair, bleaches strip the hair of its own color and since it's possible to bleach hair to varying degrees of blondeness, it's best to consult a reputable hair stylist for desired results.

Semi-permanent tints, known as rinses, offer temporary color with few of the disadvantages of permanent dyes. With them, the chemical film penetrates only the hair's outer layer, and because the chemical reaction is less intense the color washes out within weeks. Experts recommend them especially to highlight natural hair shades (golden on brown hair, reddish on brown) rather than to significantly change color or cover grey hair. And because they're applied much like a shampoo (products differ in the length of time they need to be left on before being rinsed off) you can easily apply them yourself at home.

Haircuts

Hair styles are like hem lengths. Fashion, mood and personal style dictate whether they're to be long or short. Essentially, the secret to flattering hair is to choose a good stylist who'll give you the right cut as well as other relevant hair care advice. How to choose a hair stylist? Consider the following:

- Ask your friends for their recommendations as to who is good in town and why. Or, when you see someone, even a stranger, with a hair style you like, ask them where they got their hair done and by whom?

- Try to make the first appointment with a new hair stylist at a time when the salon is not frantic. This is usually mid-week, or it may be early morning. Even if it's not your best time, try to make that first appointment at a time when your hair stylist isn't too busy and can take the time to talk to you and think more clearly about what suits you.

- While it's great to go to a hair stylist relaxed, in old or casual clothes, it's also a good idea to show your hair stylist what you look like when you get your act together so that your new hair cut can better reflect the real you.

- By all means, use magazines to show your stylist the type of style you admire. But don't expect the same style to turn out the same way on your head. Trust your hair stylist's judgement to some extent.

- By the same token, many hair stylists object to clients saying, "You're the expert. Do what you want." Since it's your hair, your face and your lifestyle, give your hair stylist some guidelines: do you like short or long hair, a fringe or a side part, the newest trend or a traditional cut? Also your lifestyle: at home, is your hair wash-and-wear or do you devote time to hair grooming daily?

- Since your hair stylist isn't your dentist, it's his job to make your salon visit a comfortable one. Don't bother with one who keeps you waiting an unconscionable length of time (more than 20 minutes) or who is rude or condescending. Complain if the staff is rough on your scalp at the wash basin or keeps your wet hair dripping while they talk on the phone. If you have a time limit, tell your stylist you'd like to be out by a certain time: no one should have to spend more than two hours with a hair stylist, ever.

- Never allow yourself to be pushed into a treatment you don't really want or can't afford.

- Ask about prices before you make your appointment.

- Don't choose a hair stylist who tells you a certain style is simple to tend to when you know that, for you, it won't be. Hair stylists should be sympathetic to a client's hair problems and aware of her hair grooming limitations as well as her fashion needs.

HAIR
The Ballerina Top-Knot

As a ballerina, I learned at an early age how to do interesting things with my long hair. But the most useful style, and the style I use whenever I workout and for many of my performances, is the ballerina top-knot. Here's how it's done.

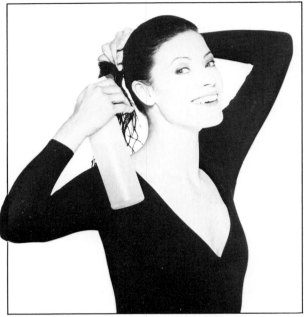

1. Pulling back my hair and grasping it at the crown, I first wet my hair, using a plastic plant-spray bottle filled with water.

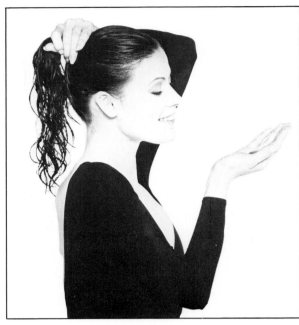

2. Instead of a hair-spray, I use a hair gel to keep my hair in place. (It also contains a conditioner.)

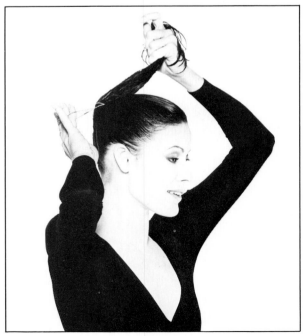

3. Using covered elastics to protect my hair, I make a pony-tail, pulling it quite tight so no hair will escape.

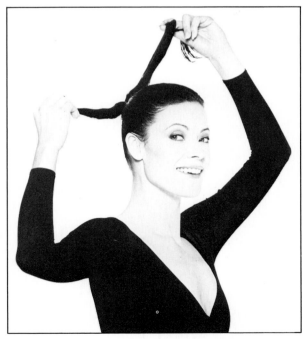

4. I split my pony-tail into two equal parts, and dividing each part further into three sections, I make a braid from each of the two parts.

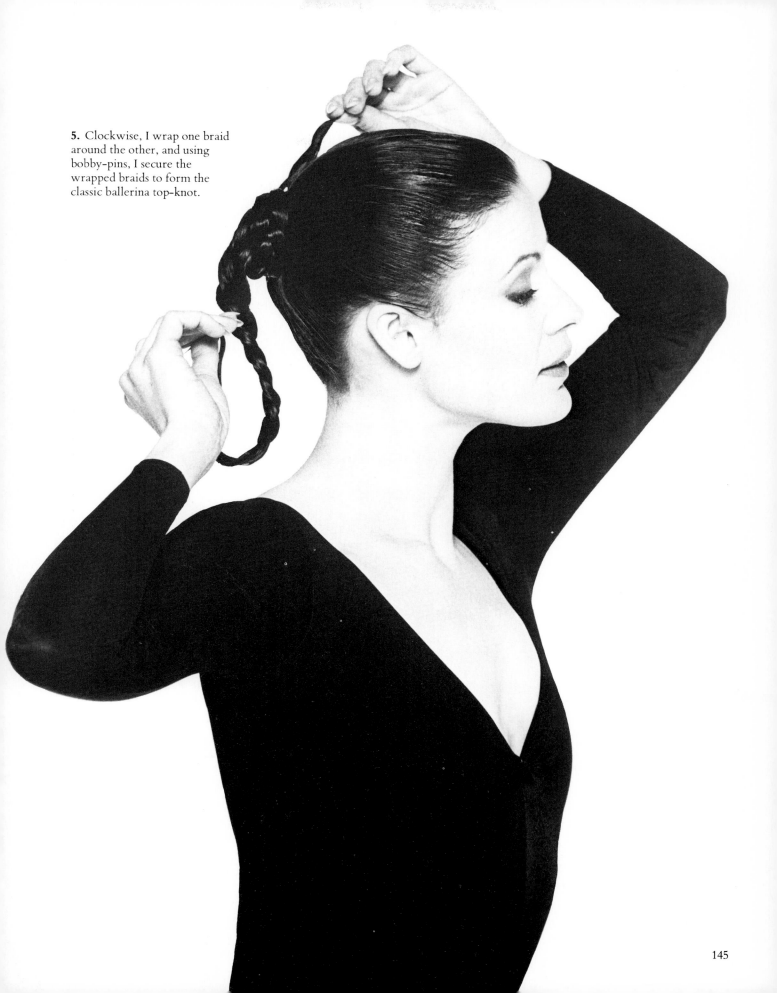

5. Clockwise, I wrap one braid around the other, and using bobby-pins, I secure the wrapped braids to form the classic ballerina top-knot.

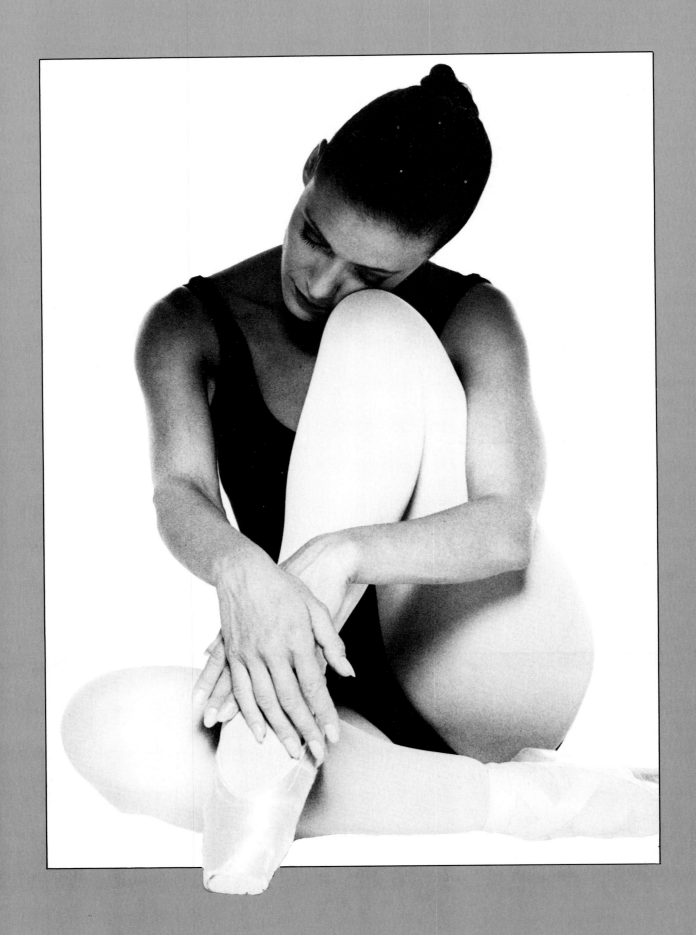

7

Feet & Hands

Feet

There's no doubt that my feet get more of a bashing than most. But since statistics show that four out of every five people eventually experience foot problems, even non-dancers are not spared the aches, pains, sprains and an assortment of other foot ailments that plague us throughout our adult years.

The trouble is, our feet were originally designed to carry one-quarter of our body weight. When you consider that, on the average, we walk the equivalent of four times around the world in a lifetime, is it any wonder that the first thing many of us do to relax is put up our feet?

But experts also say that, despite what nature gave us, most of us hinder rather than help our feet. Women, in particular, abuse their feet constantly by choosing ill-fitting shoes that tip our bodies forward, pinch our toes and, depending on the height of the heel, put undue stress on the balls of the feet. (Wearing a heel that's more than 2½ inches can strain the big toe joint, put excess pressure on the ball of the foot and even cause bunions.)

Because our feet are generally covered up, few of us care for them as much as we tend to other parts of our body—out of sight being out of mind, it seems. As well, many of us turn to our local druggist for foot care aids (plasters, pads, powders, linaments and lotions) preferring, in many instances, home care rather than care by a professional. Today, this is changing somewhat as more podiatrists set up practice. (A podiatrist, though not a physician, has had four years of training in an accredited college of podiatry and is capable of treating most foot problems as training includes learning not only about the foot's 26 bones and assorted muscles, joints, ligaments, sweat glands and blood vessels but also about all aspects of foot care. Foot problems that are major as opposed to minor are usually referred to an orthopedist, a medical doctor whose specialty includes surgery.)

While the local drug store can be of great value in providing many foot care products, there are some foot ailments you shouldn't tackle on your own. Check the following mini-guide to common foot problems in order to better judge when to seek professional care.

Ingrown Toenails

With this troublesome, often painful condition, the nail grows inward and downward into the flesh on either side of the nail, especially the big toe's nail. The sharp nail pushing into the tender skin makes the skin inflamed and sometimes infection follows. Toe-pinching shoes or cutting toenails improperly are the most common causes of this condition.

Choosing shoes with enough room for your toes will also prevent other foot problems. In nail-cutting, the mistake most of us make is in cutting the toenail the same way we file our fingernails—on an angle down into the sides. Always cut toenails straight across.

To tackle an ingrown toenail at home, soak your feet in warm soapy water for 15 minutes, then try to gently lift the imbedded nail with a Q-tip or cotton-wrapped orange stick. People with blood-circulation problems, diabetics and anyone whose ingrown toenail is red and inflamed, should seek professional help.

Brittle or Split Toenails

Some experts warn that brittle or split toenails may be indicative of medical conditions such as diabetes while others say that diet or even fluoridated water may also be the cause. If conditions persist, seek a medical opinion. Since brittle nails are difficult to cut dry, soaking the foot first is recommended.

Fallen Arches

Like the spine's slipped disc which doesn't really slip, arches don't fall. Rather, the weight of the body, due to the strained muscles that form the arch of the foot, is taken up by the flattened arch instead of by the toes and heel. Signals of fallen arches (also called flat feet) include aching feet and soreness felt up the ankle, leg and back. A podiatrist may recommend specific foot exercises for fallen arches or the use of a simple shoe inlay, or, in severe cases, a special appliance such as a brace or a band. Wooden exercise sandals sometimes alleviate the condition as do shoes made with particular attention to their arch supports.

Athlete's Foot

No doubt the term is a carry-over from the days when athletes were considered a breed apart from the rest of society. Athlete's foot, however, affects even the most sedentary person because it's so easy to catch—though the term originated probably because the condition's culprit, fungus, thrives in moist sweaty areas such as locker rooms or around pools. The fungus infection attacks the skin between the toes and the toenail area, causing redness, itchiness and soreness. As the common fungus is infectious, you may not always be able to avoid it but you can lessen your chances of getting it by keeping your feet clean, drying in between your toes and applying talcum powder between toes. Most cases of athlete's foot can be self-treated by over-the-counter preparations. If the condition persists, however, or severely flares up, consult a doctor who may prescribe a specific antifungal agent.

Corns and Calluses

Probably the two most common feet ailments, corns and calluses are also the most easily prevented by wearing shoes that fit properly. Corns, found usually between the toes or over a toe joint, are like calluses, found usually on the soles of the feet, in that both are thickening pads of skin built up in areas of excess friction and pressure. But while both are thick and unsightly, corns are often more painful than calluses. Never cut or shave off either. Instead, in treating either at home, soak the foot first, then try gently sanding the area with a pumice stone or drug-store file made especially for this purpose. While moleskin or corn plasters, when applied to corns and calluses, can guard against further irritation, experts caution against using corn-dissolving over-the-counter medications since some, containing acid, may actually harm the skin. If conditions are severe or persist, consult a podiatrist.

Bunions

Bunions, though sometimes inherited, are also caused by wearing ill-fitting or too-tight shoes that force the toes out of alignment. Outgrowths of bone at the big toe joint, they are not only ugly but also if bursitis of the big toe joint develops, the bunion enlarges and becomes even more painful. Consult a medical doctor if you have this condition since, in some severe cases, surgery may be necessary.

Plantar's Warts

Caused by a virus, plantar's warts are contagious so walking barefoot is not a good idea. When on the soles of the feet, plantar's warts can be painful. Rather than attempting to treat this yourself, consult a medical doctor.

Aching Feet

Foot swelling, tired and aching feet are all common to any one of us who spends a lot of time on his or her feet. Even those who sit all day at work may occasionally experience these conditions, particularly in hot weather. (Feet that swell, particularly during pregnancy, should be checked out by a doctor.) Putting them up, immersing feet in a cool bath or walking around barefoot for a while are all good ways to alleviate tired aching feet. Simple foot exercises, such as rising up to your tiptoes and down again, may help the tone tired foot muscles. Or you might try picking up a pencil with your toes—this stimulates the muscles as well. To refresh aching feet, try rubbing or gently massaging them in a body lotion.

Also try a warm soapy foot bath followed by a mini home-pedicure. You'll need a large pan, warm water, one capful of dishwashing detergent, a drop of baby oil, a pumice stone, a rough towel, toenail scissors, cuticle cream, hand or body lotion, cotton balls, and nail polish.

Start by soaking the feet for 15 minutes in a large pan of warm water to which you've added the detergent and baby oil. Towel dry your feet, including in between your toes. Use a pumice stone to smooth rough spots. Gently massage in body lotion. Trim nails by cutting straight across. Apply a cuticle cream and push back cuticles gently. Separate toes with cotton balls. Apply polish. Repeat with other foot.

Hands

When you consider that hands are used to caress loved ones, to write letters, to groom ourselves, to distinguish between hot and cold or silk and mohair, and to clasp, reach, grab and pull, there's no doubt as to the importance of caring for them. And because we use them daily, in doing everything from dialing a phone to greeting a loved one, hands, probably more than any other part of the body, are subject to more wear and tear—from bumps and minor cuts to dryness from the cold.

Just immersing hands in water as much as we do is bound to dehydrate them. Add any soap, dish detergent or cleaning liquid and our hands are further assaulted, our skin defatted. All the more reason to keep hand lotion close by any sink or to wear rubber gloves (though not for longer than ten minutes at any one time) when tackling any serious cleaning job. Mild soap, a little lemon juice added to stained patches of skin, and cloth gloves worn while gardening are other ways of protecting the hands from everyday abuse. As with the face, moisturization is the key. Ironic as it sounds, the more our hands are in water, the thirstier they get.

Unlike our feet, backs or necks, it's rare to experience fatigue in the hands. But while we rarely hear ourselves complain, "Oh, my aching hands!" it's interesting to observe the reaction we have to our hands being massaged. Try it. Chances are, you'll experience a lovely feeling of relaxation, of well-being. If you're the least bit arthritic, you may find that massaging one hand with the other coupled with immersion in a warm water bath is heavenly. To massage your hand, grasp the palm and back of your left hand with the thumb and fingers of your right hand and knead gently. Then, using the thumb and forefinger of your right hand, firmly stroke each finger of your left hand working from the knuckle to the fingertip.

Having a professional manicure now and then is one of the nicest things you can do for yourself as well as for your nails. In having it done, you're forced to relax—it's difficult even to read while one hand is plopped into soapy water—and your nails, in the end, have a neat sparkling look that is virtually impossible to achieve on your own (unless, of course, you're ambidextrous).

But even if you can't achieve a truly professional shape and shine on your own, it's well worth trying a home manicure to keep your nails in shape, healthy looking and clean.

For a basic home manicure, you'll need the following: cotton balls, an emery board or two, an orange stick, a bowl of warm water to which a drop of baby oil and a capful of mild dishwashing detergent has been added, a cuticle cream, cuticle remover, hand cream and a towel. If you wear nail polish, have the color of your choice handy. If you are wearing old nail polish, you'll need polish remover. Now, sit back comfortably at a table in an area of good light.

1. Using the emery board, file each nail into a gentle oval shape—filing from the sides toward the middle. Avoid cutting with scissors as they may split the nail. File nails after polish is removed.

2. Rub cuticle cream into the cuticle area.

3. Soak fingers in a bowl of soapy warm water to which you've added the baby oil and dish detergent.

4. Apply cuticle remover to cuticle area.

5. Using the blunt end of an orange stick wrapped in a cotton ball, push the cuticle gently down and back all round the nail.

6. Now, clean out the nail tip area with the pointed end of the orange stick wrapped in a cotton ball. (You may prefer to use a white nail crayon as well.)

7. Massage hand lotion into hand and fingers using swift strokes on each finger from the knuckle area to the nail tip.

As beautiful as polished nails are, remember that your nails, like your hair, which is also dead, reflect the general state of your health. Beware of nail grooming aids that promise instant beauty and renewed health. Like hair grooming aids, their effects will be purely cosmetic.

Proper nail care and attention to good health principles will prevent the following common problems, too:

Split or Brittle Nails

These may be signs of emotional stress or may be caused by subjecting the hands to too much water and detergent. Because the nail is dead, gelatin supplements or nourishing creams, contrary to belief, won't alleviate these conditions. Best to tend to your split or brittle nails with manicures, then wait about three and a half months until the nail has a chance to grow out completely to see if the condition has changed.

White Spots on Nails

No, these are not like tea leaves whose shapes and placements may be read as signs of your emotional or physical state. Chances are they're caused by general wear and tear—bangs or knocks to the matrix or root of the nail. Polish covers them up. And they grow out with time.

Hangnails

These can be painful and are always unsightly. But since they're nothing but tiny tears in the cuticle and surrounding skin, they can be helped somewhat by applying a cuticle cream and keeping the cuticle trimmed.

Bitten Nails

Some people reach for a cigarette or a cookie. Others bite their nails. Habits, as we all know, are difficult to break, and the difficulty with breaking one habit is that the next one to replace it could be worse. Nail biting can be discouraged, however, by having regular manicures (Do you dare nibble at those beautiful nails you paid someone to do for you?) or by applying a commercial ill-tasting anti-biting deterrent. False nails are also an answer to ugly bitten nails.

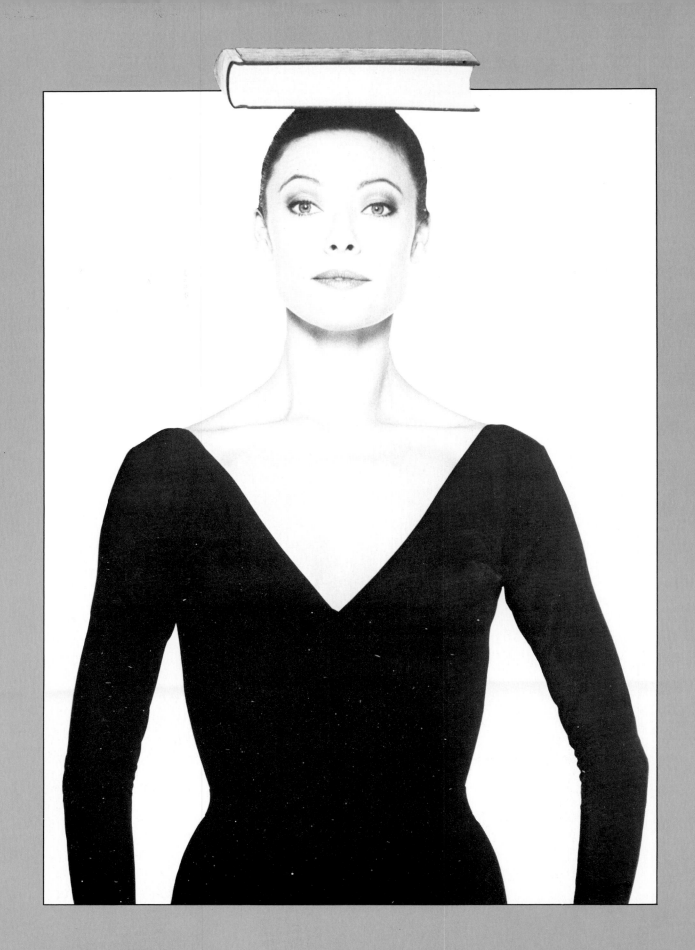

8

Posture

Posture

Bad posture is the enemy of us all. In childhood and adolescence, it is the source of a mother's constant nagging to straighten up. In later life, it can lead to nagging of a different sort—nagging backache. If we are truly interested in changing our appearance and the way in which others perceive us, one of the most visible and immediate changes can be made by standing taller. You know yourself that when it comes to body language, you receive a much different impression from someone who carries himself erect and proudly than you do from someone who slouches into a room showing all the spine of an earthworm.

In some ways, bad posture is a matter of laziness. It feels easier to slump, with the knees hyper-extended, taking the work away from muscles that would otherwise be employed keeping the body lifted and straight. But another aspect of bad posture— especially among tall women—is historic, and stems from feelings of insecurity or inferiority. In the past, the stereotype of the woman has been small, petite and vulnerable in the presence of a man. Somewhere in the past, women were led to believe that they were *supposed* to be shorter than any man who ever walked the earth—perhaps because the fragile male ego equated height with superiority and felt they could dominate shorter creatures. Hollywood perpetuated this image by standing certain leading men on orange crates so that they towered over their female co-stars. Tall women, those 5 feet 10 inches or so, always shopped for low-heeled shoes and walked with their chins buried in their chests. Fortunately, this absurd sort of self-depreciation and discrimination has largely been eradicated. Now, our top models are all tall women and tall actresses have made height extremely fashionable.

Yet even now, when it is socially acceptable to stand tall, few of us in North America do so. We spend the day bending over desks or over housework, stand with a slouch, sprawl exhausted at the end of the day into overstuffed, non-supportive chairs, and then wonder why our backs hurt. Our spines and back muscles were not meant to take this sort of abuse. We are supposed to stand erect. Isn't that what separates us from hairier primates?

North Americans, especially, seem to have something against walking with their heads held high. They're afraid to stand out. They think it makes them appear to be snobbish or affected. They shuffle down the street, refusing to make eye contact, staring down as though they expect at any moment to have their ankles mugged.

"This doesn't happen in Europe," notes my chiropractor, David Drum of Toronto. "People there aren't afraid to stand upright and look a little aristocratic. They're nationalistic and proud, and it's reflected in the way they carry themselves."

David further observes that it is precisely this type of upright carriage that sets dancers apart from everyone else when they walk into a room. Without vanity, I have to admit that it feels good when people notice me. David believes strongly that it is this striking, visual first impression that dancers convey—having a slightly regal air because of their uprightness—that is one of the attractions of ballet.

Small wonder that when some patients go to doctors or chiropractors with postural problems, the exercise prescription often given is for a routine of ballet-type training. Years of this training and the consequent development of muscles in the lower back and abdomen has been found to help flatten out the curve of the lower spine, reducing stress and adding slightly to one's perceived height.

Continually forced to keep the body upright against gravity, our spines assume stresses that are quite considerable. Consider the spine's structure, for example. Instead of being built like a tower of blocks, one firmly set on top of the other, the spine's 24 small circular bones are arranged in an S-curve—a modern engineering miracle or a disaster, depending on how you look at it. Each vertebra, resting on the one below it at an angle, depends on surrounding muscles and ligaments to hold it there. Awkward posture, or muscle strain through overwork, strains the muscular support system and causes debilitating backache. Each of the vertebra is separated by cartilage shock-absorbers, known as discs. They are designed to protect the sensitive spine and the spinal cord that passes through it, by absorbing the impact of body weight during movement. If the surrounding muscles lose their strength, the rim of the spinal disc weakens and tears, allowing part of its gelatinous centre to herniate—pressing painfully on nerve tissue.

Properly treated, the back does not have to be as unstable as the physiological description makes it sound. It is a multi-piece structure, which if kept flexible and well-supported by muscles is designed to allow us a very wide range of movement. Part of back health evolves from common sense. Bending at the waist to lift an object is unwise. The vertebrae move apart at the rear, pinch at the front and the muscles around them are being asked to do all the work. It is far wiser to lift from a squatting position (however inelegant), with the back kept straight. This way, the large, load-bearing muscles of the thighs can do most of the lifting. Pulling a heavy object, such as a table, is kinder to the back than pushing it. Your arms and shoulders accept some of the load in pulling, whereas in pushing the force gets transferred to the spine and compresses the discs. Carrying a heavy package should be done with the parcel clutched close to the body, where it can be close to the centre of gravity and balanced over the feet and legs. To carry it with arms outstretched creates a much more radical shift in one's centre of gravity, perhaps to a point outside the body, and taxes the back muscles.

If you keep the back healthy—and we include some strengthening and flexibility exercises in this section—good posture can become a matter of practice, then a natural habit. First off, let's get rid of the myth that good posture is the bolt-upright military stance with the hips forward, shoulders back and chest thrust out. This arches the spine in a backward curve; it doesn't represent a straight back at all. At the other end of the spectrum, neither is Venus de Milo a model to be copied. She may be famous the world over as a symbol of beauty and grace, but she has one shoulder dipped and one hip thrust forward. If she had a spine, it would be a spiral or a double-S—one S traceable in cross-section from front to back, the other from left to right.

Think of good posture as being achieved by imagining a steel rod passing through your body, head to foot, at these points: from the top middle of your head, to just behind the ears, to behind the shoulder joints, down through the sacrum, through the knee joints and down through the calf to the foot, in front of the ankle. If you were standing against a wall, the back of the head, apex of the thoracic spine, buttocks and heels would all be in line, touching the wall. Natural curves in the spine would allow for gaps between the wall and the back of the neck and in the small of the back.

No one stands this way constantly, but by constantly reminding yourself, you can naturally develop the muscles needed to keep this posture more and more of the time. Understand further that posture is not a static thing, but dynamic. We are, by nature, mobile creatures and we have to work at proper, upright carriage during walking as well as while standing or sitting.

David Drum mentions in his *Introduction to the Study of Spinal and Postural Mechanics* a well-known concept among back experts. It states that the closest analogy to the human body is a system of three pyramids, with their bases uppermost, balanced one on top of the other. The pelvis and legs form the lowest pyramid. The shoulders form the base of the middle inverted pyramid, with its apex situated at the lumbosacral joint. The third pyramid is the head, balanced on the cervical vertebrae in the middle of the base formed by the shoulders. Man has a high centre of gravity, with most of his mass located in the chest and stomach area. According to laws of physics, this should make us precariously unstable creatures.

It takes constant work to keep these balance points relatively in line during movement, but deviation from it takes away from ease of movement and requires us to use energy to keep correcting balance, whether we recognize it or not. David Drum quotes Dr. Lyman Johnson, a guru among back experts, in stating that to correct faulty postural patterns, a patient must learn a new point of balance. This is not an easy matter. Experience has demonstrated to David that it is nearly impossible to establish postural re-education in a patient suffering from chronic fatigue. He cites H. G. McCormick's hypothesis of 1942 that the energy cost of a slouching posture—with knees hyperextended as completely as the joints permit, hips pushed forward and head drooping—is minimal. It conserves energy in a static position. For these people to put forth more energy when their reserve is already low is a difficult proposition.

Posture while sleeping is equally important. We can achieve the best rest when the back is in its most comfortable position. If you are large or round in the buttocks, it can happen that your lower back is actually up off the mattress while you sleep on your back. A good way to remedy this, and to promote the pelvic tilt (shown in this section), which is a foundation of good posture, is to place a pillow under the knees when lying on the back. It rolls the lower back into a flat position, taking stress off the muscles and discs and allowing for more complete rest. (Remember to use the pelvic tilt when upright, as well.) Sleep on a firm mattress, with a single pillow under the head, rather than two, to avoid stretching out the muscles in the back of the neck.

Because firm abdominal muscles are a must for a good figure and good posture, sit-ups of a sort will be necessary. The type recommended by David Drum are called abdominal "crunches." I refer to them, in my five exercises for the back, as gentle sit-ups. Lie on the floor with the back as flat as possible, pressing the low back down. The knees should be up, with the soles of the feet flat on the floor. Tuck your chin to your chest and slowly start to raise your upper body, a little at a time. Try to feel each vertebra as it comes off the floor. Sit up about half to three-quarters of the way, then slowly roll back down.

The gentle back stretch is a flexibility exercise, designed to alternately stretch out and flex the muscles through the back area. Remember that all muscles need to be stretched out when they have been worked. The seated arch is part of what David Drum refers to as chair-dancing. Again, flexibility is the aim. Chair-dancing is what we might call squirming and fidgeting among children. Sitting for long periods can become highly uncomfortable and fatiguing because of the stress it puts on us. We can alleviate some of this and make the chair less of a restraint device by contracting our buttocks, shifting frequently and sitting with our feet supported slightly off the floor. The fifth exercise, the gentle twist, is geared toward freeing the articulations or swivel points in the spine.

Among exercises that might be avoided is old-fashioned toe-touching from a standing position. This form of flexibility training for back and hamstrings can be practiced by sitting, legs out on the floor, and stretching forward toward the toes. Straight-leg situps are no longer advised as a tummy strengthener, because it makes the hip-flexors (illiopsoas muscles) pull against the lower back. Use the crunches, instead. Chest-raises, while lying face down, are similarly not advised because they can be very hard on the untoned back of a beginner and dangerous for those with unstable backs.

FIVE EXERCISES FOR THE BACK
The Right Way and the Wrong Way

When you are doing exercises that involve lying on your back, be sure to push the small of your back into the floor like this.

Don't arch it like this.

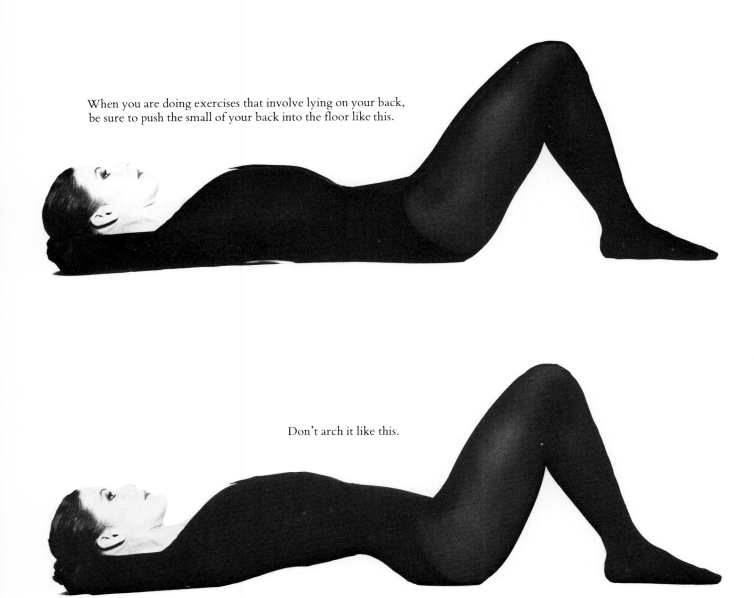

These five exercises soothe and strengthen the back without putting extra strain on it. Even if you have a back problem, pay special attention to the pelvic tilt when doing sit-ups or other abdominal exercises. And before you try any of these exercises, here or elsewhere, consult a doctor.

1. Lie on the floor with your knees bent. Place your right or left hand beneath the small of your back, palm down on the floor. Feel each vertebra pressing against the floor.

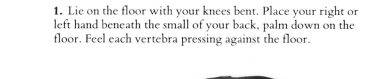

2. By contracting your stomach muscles and squeezing your buttocks muscles, press your back into your hand. Relax and repeat as often as you need to in order to understand this technique.

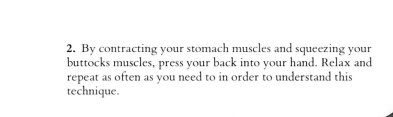

3. Now, do the pelvic tilt again, but this time place your arms under your head, and slowly slide both legs out on the floor in front of you. Be sure to keep the small of the back pressed into the floor. Repeat six times.

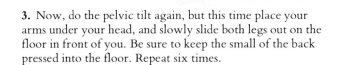

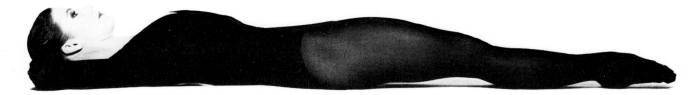

FIVE EXERCISES FOR THE BACK

2. The Gentle Sit-Ups

Very often, a weak back is due to weak stomach muscles, but when you try to strengthen your stomach muscles you may hurt your back. To break this circle of frustration, work on the following—an easy-on-your-back exercise that begins to strengthen the abdominals while it relieves strain on the back.

1. Lie on your back, knees bent, arms relaxed at your sides.

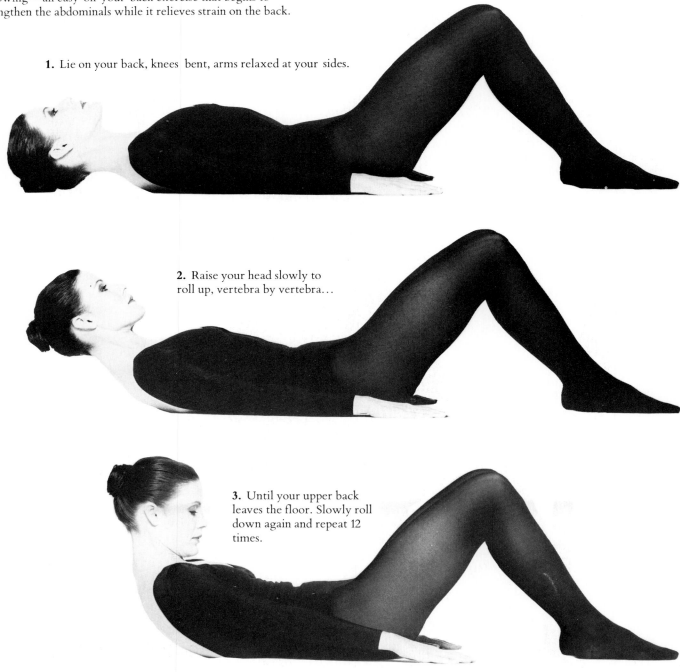

2. Raise your head slowly to roll up, vertebra by vertebra...

3. Until your upper back leaves the floor. Slowly roll down again and repeat 12 times.

3. The Seated Arch

This is one back exercise you can do at the office, on a long airplane flight, or wherever you can find a seat—it's great for relieving tension during a hectic day.

1. Find a chair with a long seat so you can sit comfortably, not precariously, on the edge. Sit up straight, hands on knees, feet flat on the floor. Press your lower back forward and upward trying to lengthen the spine and lift the chest to the ceiling—arching your back slightly.

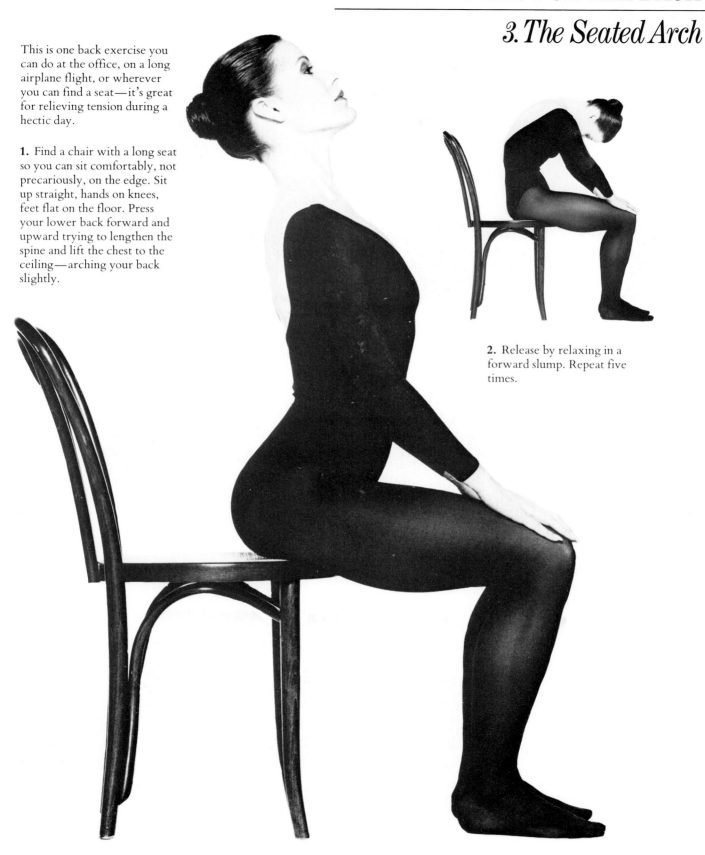

2. Release by relaxing in a forward slump. Repeat five times.

FIVE EXERCISES FOR THE BACK

4. The Gentle Back Stretch

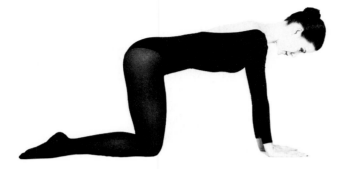

1. Get onto your hands and knees, hands about shoulder distance apart, knees about hip distance apart.

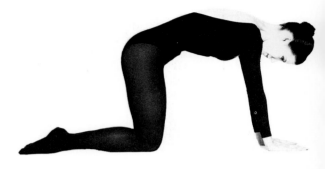

2. Begin to round your back, starting with the lower back...

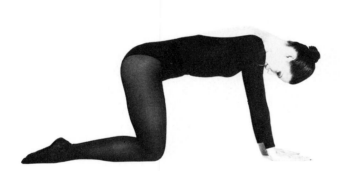

4. Now begin to release the movement by straightening out your back.

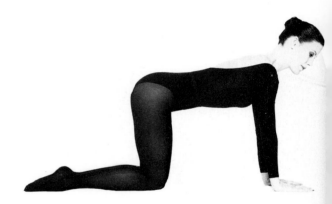

5. Then, arch your back beginning with the lower part of your back...

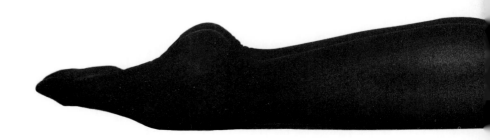

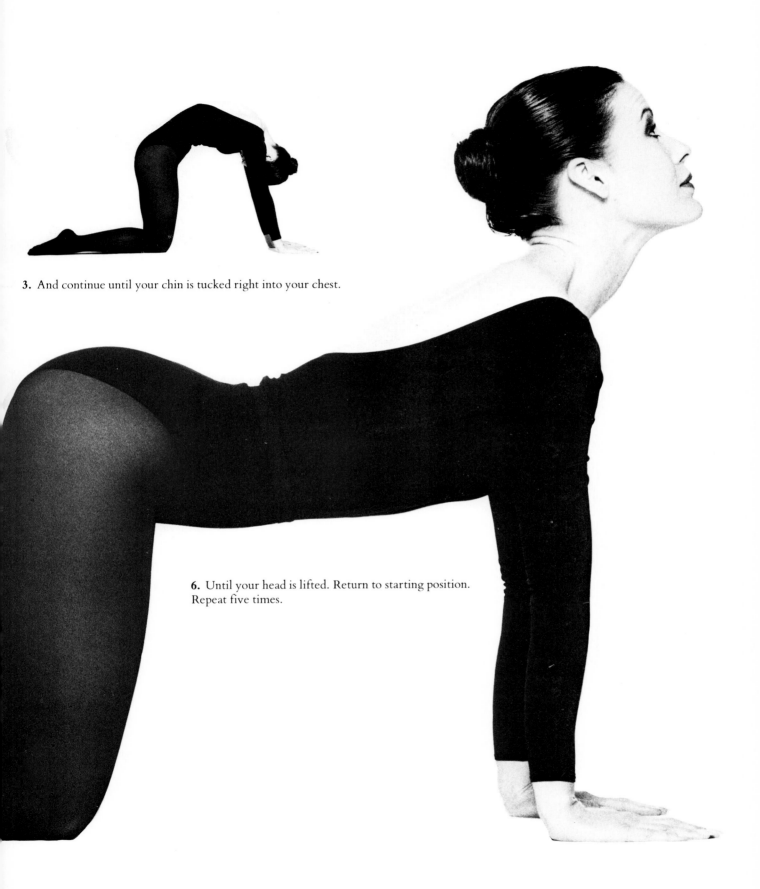

3. And continue until your chin is tucked right into your chest.

6. Until your head is lifted. Return to starting position. Repeat five times.

FIVE EXERCISES FOR THE BACK

5. The Gentle Twist

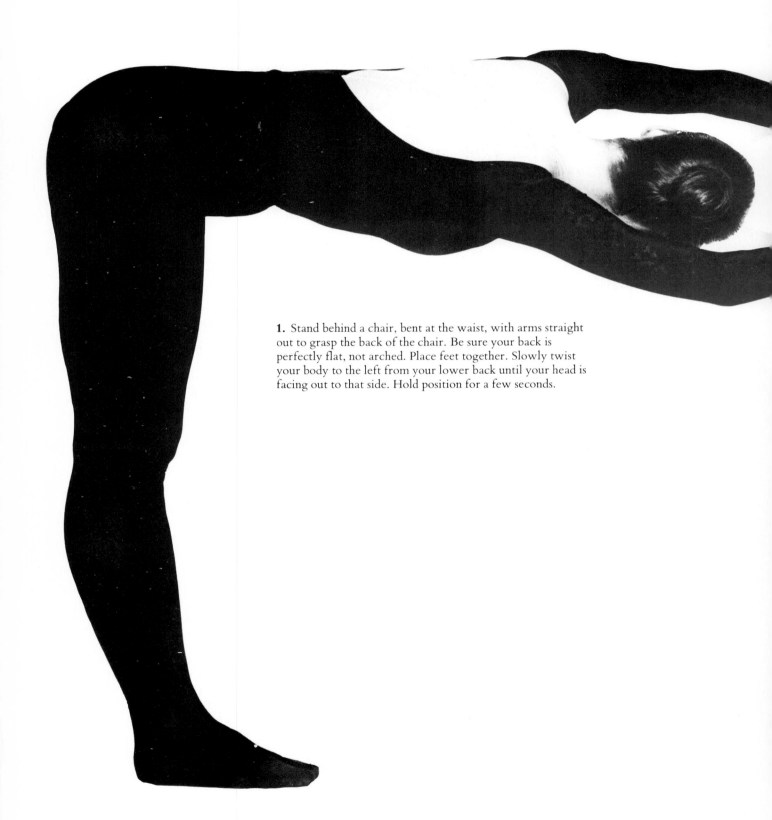

1. Stand behind a chair, bent at the waist, with arms straight out to grasp the back of the chair. Be sure your back is perfectly flat, not arched. Place feet together. Slowly twist your body to the left from your lower back until your head is facing out to that side. Hold position for a few seconds.

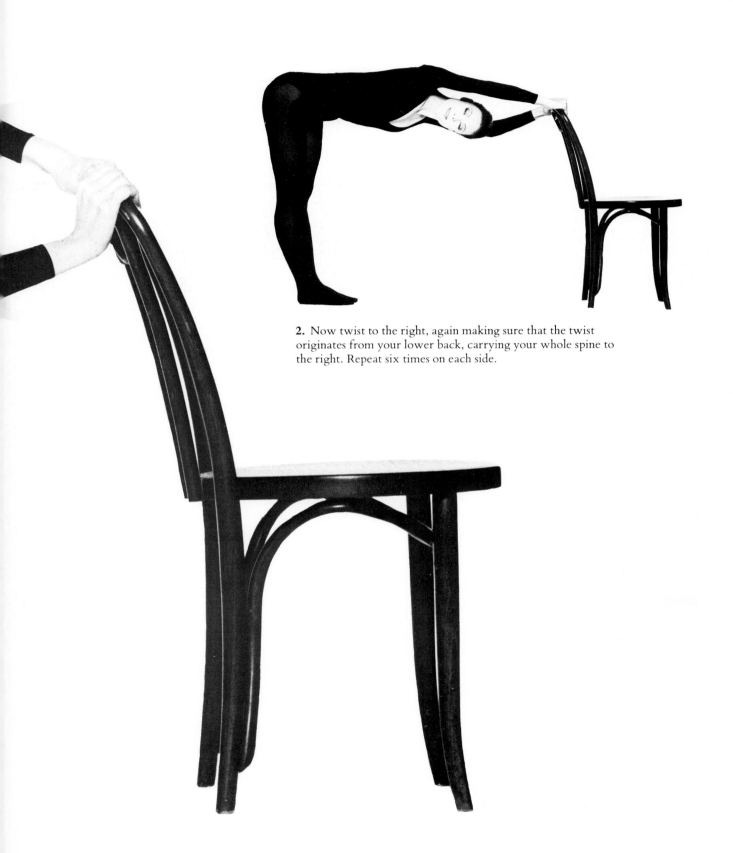

2. Now twist to the right, again making sure that the twist originates from your lower back, carrying your whole spine to the right. Repeat six times on each side.

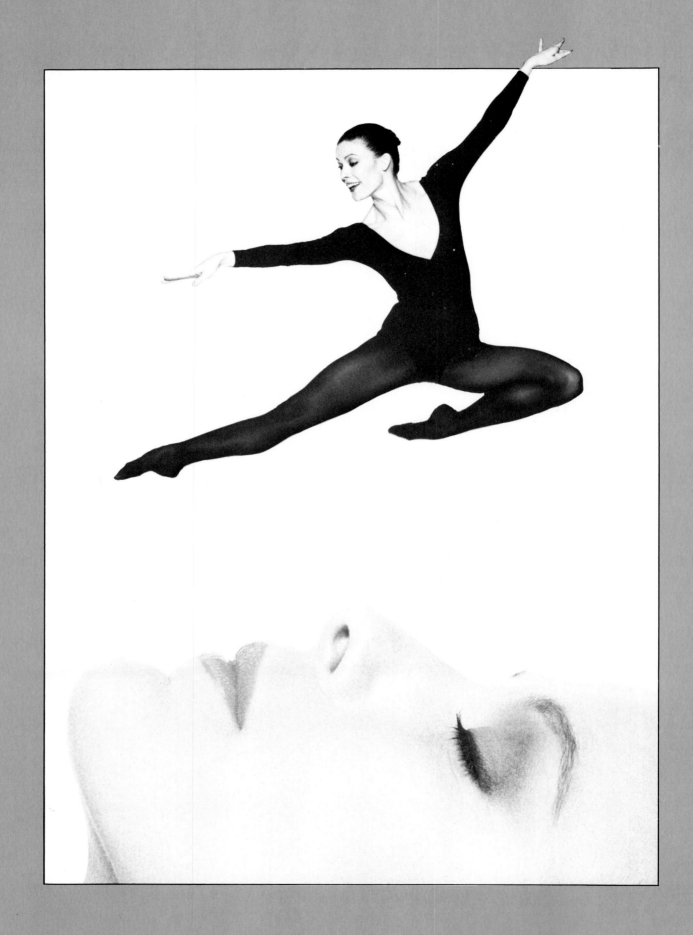

9

Sleep & Relaxation

Sleep

Like the food we eat and the air we breathe, sleep is absolutely vital to life. It's the one-third of our lives that most affects the other two. It recharges our batteries, prepares us to meet the next day's challenges. No matter what it is we each do during our waking hours, sleep is something we all have to do.

But how much sleep is enough? Woodrow Wilson needed nine straight hours a night. Napoleon, only three. I find that I have to have at least eight hours every night.

Between seven and nine hours is what most people say when asked how much sleep they think they need. The proper amount of sleep is something everyone has to figure out for themselves, and the best way to do that is simply to experiment.

Start with the number of hours you think you need (six, for example) and try to ensure that, for three straight weeks, you get six hours nightly. Then, take note of how you feel after this time. If you're drowsy and listless (particularly about 3 P.M.—when the mid-afternoon "slump" sets in), try the next three weeks on seven hours a night. If you feel energized and rested on six, however, you may need less sleep than you thought.

I know how good I feel when I get enough sleep, but I still resist getting myself into bed early enough sometimes. Early to bed and early to rise are not always a part of my lifestyle. After a performance, I'm really pretty wound up. I go to sleep about 3 A.M., but then I let myself sleep in. Late-night performances combined with the stresses of jet lag mean that my sleep cycle can become disrupted, often.

But I'm lucky that I'm a napper. Get me on a bus and in twenty minutes I'm gone. If I have four hours in an airport, I can catch a nap. It's typical to find dancers catnapping on the floor while rehearsal takes place around them. And I can sometimes be found sleeping in my dressing room while waiting for my next rehearsal to begin. A dancer's life is demanding, exciting and exhausting. When you're really physically tired, it's easy to fall asleep!

But every second person in North America has suffered from occasional bouts of insomnia, and, when faced with travel time changes, I'm no exception. "If you can't sleep, try lying on the end of the bed—then you might drop off," Mark Twain advised, tongue firmly in cheek. Napoleon believed that his feet pointing north would assure sound sleep. For Charles Dickens, going to bed with his head pointed north was important. Of course, I don't care which way my head or feet are pointing. Here are some tried and true tips on getting to sleep:

1. Toes to Nose: Complete Relaxation

This old trick works for most people who try it. Settle yourself into bed, then begin by concentrating on relaxing only your toes. Then, relax your whole left foot followed by your right foot. Moving up your body, relax every limb and muscle one by one. Do this inch by inch until you melt right into the bed, and by the time you get to your nose, chances are you'll be asleep.

2. Soft Gentle Tunes

During the day, choose some favorite music—that is, relaxing tunes, not rock 'n'roll. Have the tape or record player near you at bedtime and allow the music to become part of your going to sleep ritual.

3. Move, but Don't Exercise

One time when you don't exercise is just before you go to bed—you'll feel too perky to sleep. Doctors do recommend more exercise during the day, however, to help you sleep better at night. If you find your sleep disrupted or if you can't fall asleep after an hour, don't lie there fretting and tossing and turning. Get up, go to another room and return to bed when you're drowsy. Or, turn on your night-light and read.

4. Have a Cuppa

I have a cup of linden tea as well as other herbal varieties before going to bed. Stay away from coffee or tea, both of which contain caffeine, a stimulant. If you don't care for herbal teas or decaffeinated teas, try a banana or a cup of warm milk, each of which contain the substance tryptophan, a natural relaxant. Or buy some L-Tryptophan at the health food store. I often use it when I'm nervous the night before a big performance.

5. Think Calm Thoughts

Imagine the first snowfall, a mountain stream, a clear cool lake or a perfect rose garden. Try to visualize not only this perfect setting but also yourself in it. Unclench your fists, lightly close your eyes. Or, try the old trick of counting sheep, or counting backwards from 100. Sounds corny, but it really can work. James Thurber spelled words backwards to tempt sleep. Another of his tricks was to rewrite Poe's "The Raven"—but from the bird's point of view.

6. Find a Soothing Ritual

Russia's Catherine the Great, plagued by insomnia, had her hair brushed every night to relax before bed. A long lazy soak in a bubble bath also helps. So does a full-body light massage with your favorite non-greasy body lotion.

7. Check out the Environment

Make sure the climate of your bedroom is conducive to sleeping. During winter, our rooms may get too dry and too hot. A humidifier and a turned-down thermostat help. Sleep studies show that we sleep best at temperatures between 64° and 68°F. And make sure your mattress is comfortable. There should be no sinking at the centre, no sign of lumps when you lie on it. Doctors agree that a firm mattress is best. Too hard and you'll get pain in your shoulders and hips; too soft, and you'll be plagued with lower back pain.

If you've ever tried to keep awake during school when studying for exams or even during an all-night dance marathon, you'll remember how difficult it was to fight the sandman. There are various theories about why we need to sleep at all. But since sleep research, unlike sleep itself, is less than fifty years old, there's no definitive answer. Suffice to say that sleep represents renewal for our bodies and that, deprived of sleep, we suffer.

It used to be thought that, once asleep, our bodies were completely at rest having passed from one state of consciousness to another coma-like state. But recent research has concluded that we pass through a series of four sleep stages.

In stage one, usually lasting about ten minutes, we move from being awake into a light slumber, which is represented by a slowing down process: a drop of body temperature, a lessening of pulse rate, slower breathing and a change in brain waves.

In stage two, lasting about 25 minutes, the eyeballs begin to move under the eyelids as our brain waves increase in frequency; we are moving deeper into sleep.

Stage three, total relaxation, is marked by a further drop in temperature and blood pressure. And with stage four, deep sleep, our brain waves show up large and slow-moving when measured on an electroencephalograph. Throughout each night, we repeat these four stages of sleep four or five times.

But sleep is more complex still. During certain sleep stages, we experience rapid eye movement patterns (REM) in which our eyes dart back and forth under our lids. This REM sleep brings with it certain physiological changes such as irregular breathing and an increase in heartbeat. Though our brain waves during this phase resemble those at waking, it is during REM that we dream the most.

REM sleep, in fact, is a key to understanding why some of us wake up refreshed after five hours sleep and others feel weary or fuzzy after nine. Studies in which sleeping subjects are deprived of REM sleep (when their eyelids begin to flicker, they are woken up) indicate that when deprived of this stage of sleep we become tense and irritable in the morning. Research has furthermore shown that poor sleepers spend less time in this REM state than so-called healthy sleepers. Sleeping pills and alcohol also interfere with the REM phase.

Relaxation

Relaxation is just as important as sleep in maintaining sound health. To be a dancer, you have to be disciplined, not just with exercise but with time. I find I have to block time for myself—whether or not I'm going off on a holiday. I can work hard, right through weekends if necessary, as long as I know I'm going to have time to recuperate.

Your own prescription for relaxation is something you have to write for yourself. I love to go to movies or read magazines to relax. Sometimes I'll go to a cafe or lie in the sun to read. Or I get a long book, a good biography or historical fiction, and get so involved that I won't be able to put it down.

But relaxation can also come from a good workout. Fitness clubs report that their busiest hours are at the end of the work day.

The fact is that few of us are ever free from the tensions of everyday life—job deadlines, monthly budgets, cars that sometimes quit or clogged kitchen sinks. When super stresses are added to these everyday annoyances, however, tension really mounts. To measure serious stresses, two stress experts, Dr. Thomas Holmes and Dr. Richard Rahe, developed a list of 43 major events that may occur in an adult's life to cause varying degrees of stress. By assigning a rating to each event, they concluded that it's possible to measure a person's stress.

Try giving yourself the Holmes-Rahe stress test by circling the following life events that apply to you and adding up the relevant numbers.

Life Event	Value
1. Death of spouse	100
2. Divorce	73
3. Marital separation	65
4. Jail term	63
5. Death of close family member	63
6. Personal injury or illness	53
7. Marriage	50
8. Fired from job	47
9. Marital reconciliation	45
10. Retirement	45
11. Change in health of family member	44
12. Pregnancy	40
13. Sex difficulties	39
14. Gain of new family member	39
15. Business readjustment	39
16. Change in financial state	38
17. Death of close friend	37
18. Change to different line of work	36
19. Change in number of arguments with spouse	35
20. Mortgage over $10,000 (this might be higher now)	31

If your stresses prove to be medium (200 to 299) or severe (300 or more), take time to teach your body the language of relaxation. Relaxation is an important antidote to stress, which, when prolonged, may contribute to ulcers or even heart disease. Many people seek refuge in alcohol or drugs to deal with stress but better you should try the following anti-stress tips instead.

1. A Quick Pick-me-up

Get some fresh air, even if it's only five minutes worth. Take five slow, deep breaths, holding each breath for the count of six and letting each out as slowly as possible.

2. Lie Down, Stretch Out, Curl Up

Granted, this isn't easy to do when you're working in an office. But you can take five minutes to close your eyes on the couch at home after work and before an evening out. If you're worried about falling asleep and missing your dinner date, set the timer for 10 to 20 minutes.

3. Relax at your Desk

Sit up straight. Keep your shoulders straight but slowly roll your head in a circle round your neck, five times clockwise. Then repeat, counterclockwise. Take three deep slow breaths. Now, hunch both shoulders forward, then relax them. Repeat five times.

4. A Change is as Good as a Rest

To help relax, I often ride my bike—not exactly rest for a dancer, but relaxation, nonetheless. Try gardening, knitting, photography or contact your local YWCA to find out about the classes offered. Or get to know your local library and become your own expert through reading. Anything you choose to do can provide temporary relief from everyday stresses, providing you make time for it. I find that it helps a lot to find a day when I can simply tune out the world. I unplug the phone, don't open my mail and leave the newspapers to be read one morning in bed. Another good idea would be to check into a hotel for a weekend or look for a special spa package—three days of exercise, massage and all-out pampering.

5. Simplify your Life

Often, we can't relax because we feel that too much is expected of us. But sometimes, we're the ones who set up the hurdles to jump. Knowing our limitations, in energy and time, can prevent us from getting on a treadmill. What can you do once you're on and want to get off? I make a list of my priorities; then, I list the things I've set out for myself to do. Sometimes I end up cutting my lists by half—at least until I'm better able to cope and have found a way to ensure more time for myself. We all have to make the time to relax, give it to ourselves and make sure we get some at least once a week. Find your best work/relax ratio and stick to it!

6. Try Yoga

A series of postures rather than exercises form the basis of yoga, an ancient philosophy rooted in Indian mystical thoughts. Its supporters maintain that regular practice promotes a tranquility that makes one less vulnerable to everyday stresses. Yoga courses are offered regularly through YWCAs and community centres. The art of physical and mental control is one that's easy to learn, though difficult to master, and can be done by anyone (regardless of age and level of fitness) virtually anywhere.

7. A Body Perk-up

Take a whirlpool bath—great for relieving aches and pains and for melting away the stresses that make your body tense and tight. Or make an appointment for a facial, a manicure or pedicure. To do any of these things, you'll have to break your stress pattern. And pampering yourself a bit is just what you and your body needs from time to time. Or, you might try having a massage. If you've had one, you well know the restorative qualities it offers. You just feel so good all over. For my body, I like the good old Swedish massage—an athletic touch, not a tickle!

Having a good massage depends on finding a person trained in massage techniques who also has a sound knowledge of muscle groups and physiological structure. (Remember, a good massage, while enjoyable, doesn't subtract pounds or tighten sagging muscles. That takes exercise and diet!) Look in the Yellow Pages to find registered massage therapists. Or enquire at a reputable health club to find out if there's a good masseuse on staff.